Vitamins:
Hype or Hope?

Vitamins:
Hype or Hope?

A Concise Guide for Determining Which Nutrients You Really Need

Pamela Wartian Smith, M.D., MPH

Healthy Living Books, Inc.
TRAVERSE CITY, MI

First printing 2004

ISBN 0-9729767-4-4
LCCN 2003112573

In memory of my father,
Charles Wartian,
who taught me to never give up
on my dreams.

ACKNOWLEDGMENTS

The wisdom of so many fine people has led me to this book. I cannot hope to name them. In thanking a few, I extend my thanks to all.

To Roger Williams and Linus Pauling who were the forerunners in the field of orthomolecular/functional medicine.

To my contemporaries, Billie Sahley, David Perlmutter, Robert Crayhon, Steven Sinatra, Alan Gaby, Jonathan Wright, Ronald Klatz, Robert Goldman, Leo Galland, Michael Schmidt, Sheri Lieberman, Mark Houston, Patrick Quillin, and Eric Braverman who have taught me so much.

To Jeffrey Bland whose brilliance not only has instructed me but has rekindled my love for medicine.

To my husband, Christopher Smith, for his enduring patience and support.

To God for always lighting my path.

DISCLAIMER

This book is not intended to provide medical advice and is sold with the understanding that the publisher and the author are not liable for the misconception or misuse of information provided. The author and Healthy Living Books shall have neither liability nor responsibility to any person or entity with respect to any loss, damage, or injury caused or alleged to be caused directly or indirectly by the information contained in this book or the use of any products mentioned. Readers should not use any of the products discussed in this book without the advice of a medical professional. The information contained in this book is designed for information and education only and is not intended to prescribe treatment.

To see a board-certified physician in your area who specializes in functional medicine, contact:

- The Institute for Functional Medicine: 1-253-858-4724 or visit them on the web at: www.fxmed.com
- The American Academy of Anti-Aging Physicians: 1-773-528-4333 or visit them on the web at: www.worldhealth.net

TABLE OF CONTENTS

The doctor of the future will give no medicine but will interest his patients in the care of the human frame, in diet, and in the cause and prevention of disease.

—Thomas A. Edison

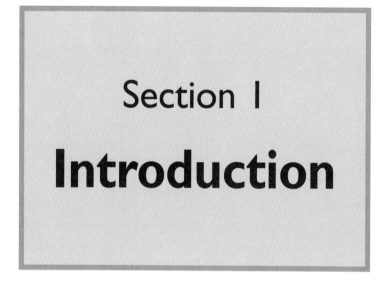

Section I

Introduction

Do you need to take vitamins and nutrients? In what amounts? Which ones? These are the questions that this book will look at answering.

The recommended daily allowances (RDAs) and the RDIs (reference daily intakes) merely serve to prevent disease. They are not designed for optimal health. The RDAs and RDIs, furthermore, do not take into account that the amount of vitamins, minerals, and other nutrients you need are different for each individual.

Almost 75 percent of your health and life expectancy is based on lifestyle, environment, and nutrition.[1] The number of years you are alive is not nearly as important as the number of years you spend healthy. Do you want to live to be 100 if you go to a nursing home at age 80? Science has shown that "not only do persons with better health habits survive longer, but in such persons, disability is postponed and compressed into fewer years at the end of life."[2] For example, a recent article in the New England Journal of Medicine examined diet, lifestyle, and the risk of type 2 diabetes mellitus in woman. The author concluded

1

that the majority of cases of type 2 diabetes could be prevented by the adaption of a healthy lifestyle.[3]

Furthermore, researchers in the Journal of the American Medical Association stated, "suboptimal vitamin states are associated with many chronic diseases including cardiovascular disease, cancer, and osteoporosis, it is important for physicians to identify patients with poor nutrition or other reasons for increased vitamin needs." They suggest that "most people do not consume an optimal amount of all vitamins by diet alone . . . it appears prudent for all adults to take vitamin supplements."[4]

Medications, vitamin interaction, soil depletion, need for more antioxidants, stress, age, lifestyle, and genetics all play a role in determining which nutrients are right for you.

To begin, the following are some examples of how medications may deplete your body of specific vitamins and minerals. Vitamins can also increase or decrease the absorption of your medications.[5]

- Long-term use of antacids (prescription or over-the-counter) can lead to decreased folic acid absorption.
- Regular use of aspirin decreases folate levels.
- Birth control pills and estrogen replacement deplete your body of B vitamins.
- Too much vitamin B6 can decrease the effectiveness of levadopa.
- Disopyramide (Norpace) and quinidine sulfate can cause magnesium deficiency.
- Colchicine reduces the absorption of beta-carotene and also possibly magnesium, potassium, and vitamin B12.
- Methotrexate decreases beta carotene, folic acid, and vitamin B12.
- Estrogen replacement increases calcium absorption.
- Seizure medications (anticonvulsants) can deplete your body of carnitine.
- H2 blockers such as cimetidine decrease vitamin D activity.

- HMG-CoA reductase inhibitors used to lower cholesterol (statin drugs) stop your body from making coenzyme Q-10.
- Medications to lower blood sugar such as glyburide (Diabeta), acetohexamide (Dymelor), and tolazamide (Tolinase) all can lead to coenzyme Q-10 deficiency.
- Digoxin can increase the rate of calcium excretion from your body.
- Fiber can decrease the absorption of digoxin.
- Diuretics (water pills) increase the loss of magnesium, potassium, sodium, and zinc.
- Calcium can decrease the absorption of beta blockers.
- Potassium-sparing diuretics deplete your body of folic acid, calcium, and zinc.

If you are on any of the above medications it is important that your doctor make sure that you replace the nutrients depleted or make sure that your vitamins and your medications do not interact.

Secondly, even the foods you eat can affect the medication you are taking. For example, be aware that grapefruit may increase the risk of side effects of the following medications:[6]

- Calcium-channel blockers (e.g., nifedipine, amlodipine, verapamil, felodipine) if taken with grapefruit can decrease blood pressure, cause flushing, headache, and increased heart rate.
- Grapefruit increases the levels of quinidine.
- Grapefruit can cause irregular heart rhythms if you are taking terfenadine.
- If you are taking a sedative (benzodiazepines, e.g., alprazolam, diazepam, midazolam, triazolam) grapefruit can increase levels of the medication.
- Grapefruit increases estrogen levels for both men and women.
- If you are taking cyclosporine, grapefruit increases the levels and can cause kidney and liver toxicity.

- Grapefruit increases the level of caffeine in your body and can cause nervousness and insomnia.
- If you are taking a macrolide antibiotic, such as clarithromycin, grapefruit will decrease its absorption.
- If you are taking fexofenadine (Allegra) grapefruit decreases the absorption of the medication.
- If you are taking statin drugs (HMG-CoA reductase inhibitors), grapefruit may increase the medication level.
- Grapefruit increases the levels of warfarin.
- Grapefruit delays the absorption of Viagra.
- Grapefruit and naprosyn taken together may cause hives.
- If you are taking carbamazepine (Tegretol), grapefruit can increase levels which may lead to nausea, tremors, drowsiness, dizziness, or agitation.
- If you are taking amiodarone, grapefruit may elevate blood levels and you may have nausea, drowsiness, tremors, or agitation.

Thirdly, vitamins and minerals, and other nutrients can also interact with each other. They do not exist in a vacuum. The nutrients have relationships and interrelationships with other nutrients. The following are examples of how vitamins and minerals interact: [7, 8, 9, 10]

- You have to have enough vitamin C in your body to use selenium effectively.
- Vitamin C can enhance the availability of vitamin A.
- Zinc in excess can decrease calcium absorption.
- Vitamin D increases the absorption of calcium and magnesium.
- Vitamin D helps your body use zinc effectively.
- Too much copper can decrease the uptake of manganese in your system.
- Vitamin A deficiency can decrease iron utilization.
- Too much iron can lower your manganese and copper levels.

- Too much riboflavin (vitamin B2) can cause magnesium deficiency.
- Vitamin B6 can cause a decrease in copper absorption.
- Vitamin A absorption may be lower if vitamin E levels are not adequate.
- Vitamin B6 deficiency can lead to a decrease use of selenium.
- Adequate phosphorus intake is needed to maintain vitamin D.

Fourthly, in today's world you cannot get all the nutrients you need from food due to the following reasons:

- The soil is deplete of many minerals such as zinc and magnesium. Selenium may be deplete or in over abundance in the ground depending on where you live. If the soil the fruits and vegetables are grown in is not rich in nutrients, then the food you eat will not contain an adequate supply of minerals.
- Fruits and vegetables begin to lose their nutritional value immediately after picking. Cold storage causes destruction of nutrients. Stored grapes lose up to 30% of their B vitamins. Tangerines stored for 8 weeks can lose almost half of their vitamin C. Asparagus stored for one week, loses up to 90 percent of its vitamin C.[11, 12]
- The nutrients in your food may not be in a form that is bioavailable. In other words, it will not be easily absorbed into your body. Orange juice is an example where 40 percent of the vitamin C in orange juice is biologically inactive.
- Processing (blanching, sterilizing, canning, and freezing) all decrease the nutritional value of the food you eat.
- The longer you cook the fruits and vegetables the less nutrients remain. Therefore, eat them raw or steamed lightly.
- The milling of grains removes 26 essential nutrients and much of the fiber.[13]

For more information concerning this subject, read *The New Nutrition* by Michael Colgan, PhD., *Dr. Art Ulene's Complete Guide to Vitamins, Minerals, and Herbs* by Art Ulene, M.D., or *The Real Vitamin and Mineral Book* by Shari Lieberman, Ph.D.

Nutritional requirements are also affected by the production of free radicals. Your body creates free radicals in many of the reactions that occur to produce energy and other substances. Free radicals are molecules that lack an electron. They will eventually rob your cells of electrons, thus damaging them. This damage contributes to oxidative stress which accelerates aging and leads to disease. In today's world, free radicals occur in the environment as well.

Causes of free radical production outside the body:

- Television screens
- Cell phones (electromagnetic fields)
- Computer screens
- Airplane trips
- Hair dryers
- Fluorescent lights
- Microwaving
- Toxic exposure to chemicals in your food, water, and air
- Excessive sunlight

When you have exposure to free radicals in the environment, your body cannot handle this extra load of oxidation. Oxidation in your body is like rust on your car. If you have extra free radicals bombarding your body all day long, your system will "rust" on the inside. Cataract formation is an example of this. In order to stop the oxidative process, you can take antioxidants which donate an electron to the free radical. This stops the destructive course.

The following are a list of some of the antioxidants that you can take:

- Vitamin A
- Vitamin C
- Vitamin E
- Selenium
- Coenzyme Q-10
- Alpha lipoic acid
- Melatonin
- Garlic
- Glutathione/NAC

Furthermore, it is paramount that antioxidants be balanced. In certain conditions too much of one antioxidant may stop the protective affects of other antioxidants.[14, 15]

Stress depletes your body of vitamins and minerals. Likewise, as you age you need more nutrients. For example, as you grow older your body makes less vitamin D, alpha lipoic acid, and less coenzyme Q-10.

Lifestyle is yet another factor that determines whether you need to take vitamins or not. If you drink alcohol it depletes your body of biotin, copper, vitamins B1, B6, B12, C and zinc. How Americans eat is also a problem since our diets are not as nutritious as they were in the past. To quote Dr. Michael Colgan in his book *The New Nutrition,* "The American diet is a major cause of disease." Lets look at a specific example.

The top 3 American vegetables eaten by children and teens are:[16]

- French fries (account for 25 percent of all vegetables consumed)
- Iceburg lettuce (99 percent water with no nutritional value)
- Ketchup (which is one-half sugar)

Adults do not fare any better. The Second National Health and Nutrition Examination (NHANES II) survey revealed:[17]

- Less than 10 percent of Americans consume 5 servings of fruits and vegetables per day
- 40 percent had no daily fruit or fruit juice
- 50 percent had no garden vegetable in a day
- 70 percent had no fruit or vegetable rich in vitamin C in a day
- 80 percent had no daily fruit or vegetable rich in carotenoids

Diet and nutritional states play a major role in influencing how your genes express themselves. Nutrients affect each step of the pathway of gene expression. As Dr. Leo Galland points out "it depends as much upon the milieu in which a gene functions as it does upon the DNA sequence of the genome."[18] In other words, even if you have inherited a gene for a particular disease such as Alzheimer's disease, whether you go on to have the disease is very much dependent on your environment, the food you eat, the toxins you are around, your stress level, and the nutrients you take in. Dr. Roger Williams discusses this situation in his book *Biochemical Individuality: The Basis for the Genotropic Concept*. He states, "Nutrition applied with due concern for individual genetic variations, which may be large, offers the solution to many baffling health problems." Your body is a lot like a car. If you put in good fuel (food and nutrients) it will run well, need little repair, and last a long time. If you put low octane fuel in your premium car (your body) your body will not run well, it will develop disease, and you will not live as long.

Many physicians say there is a lack of "peer review studies" or "scientific evidence" to show that vitamin and nutritional therapies work. To clear up this question, in 1998 alone, more than 5,000 studies were published on vitamins, more than 3,000 studies were published on antioxidants.[19] *In fact more research has been published on nutrients than on medications.*

In this book, the therapeutic techniques described are supported by hundreds of references from the literature from the most respected, peer-reviewed scientific and medical publications. These references only scratch the surface of the voluminous amount of literature that is available. To quote David Perlmutter, M.D. author of *Brain Recovery.com* and a respected neurologist: "It has been said that knowledge is power, but clearly in this context, knowledge is health."

The following sections of this book will look at vitamins, minerals, fatty acids, amino acids, and other nutrients that are used to help maintain your health and to also aid in decreasing disease. The final section of this text looks at suggested, selected, therapies that myself and other health care practitioners have used to prevent disease, to maintain optimal health, and to help treat certain disease processes.

From the above discussion you can now see that the needed number of nutrients is variable per individual. The amount of certain vitamins and minerals you may require, to promote proper functioning of your system, may be higher or less than another individual's. Dr. Linus Pauling first described this phenomena in 1968.

"Until quite recently, it was taught that everyone in this country gets enough vitamins through their diet and that taking supplements just creates expensive urine. I think we now have proof that this isn't true."

—Walter Willett, M.D.,
Harvard University

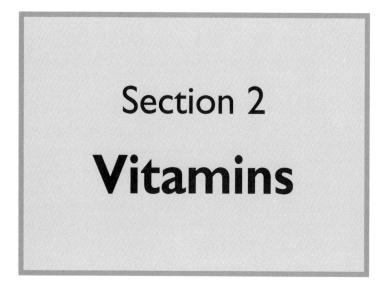

Section 2

Vitamins

Vitamins are substances that occur naturally in plants and animals. Vitamins are divided into two categories: water and fat soluble.

Fat soluble vitamins include vitamins A, D, E, K. They are stored in the fat cells of your body.

Water soluble vitamins are B and C. They are eliminated from your body the same day they are taken in.

The kind of vitamins, minerals, and nutrients you take does make a difference. The grade, form, purity, bioavailability, and third party verification, make the difference as to whether the nutrient will work for you or not.

***Vitamin supplements are divided into four quality categories:*[1]**

- Pharmaceutical grade. This grade meets the highest regulatory requirements for purity, dissolution, and absorption. There is outside verification as to the quality.
- Medical grade. This grade is a high-grade product. Prenatal vitamins usually fit into this category.

- Cosmetic, nutritional grade. Supplements of this grade may be sold in some health food stores. These often are not tested for purity, dissolution, or absorption and may not have a high concentration of the active ingredient they are labeled as.

- Feed or agricultural grade. Supplements of this grade are used for veterinary purposes. Do not take supplements of this grade.

The chemical forms of minerals are not the elemental forms. For example a 1,200 mg tablet of calcium gluconate is only nine percent elemental. This means that it only contains 108 mg of calcium. You would therefore need to take 11 capsules or tablets a day to get the recommended amount.[2]

In addition, natural or synthetic forms also makes a difference with vitamins such as vitamin E. Natural vitamin E is better absorbed and more active than synthetic.[3]

Your herbal supplements should have an adulteration screen done to see if there are any toxic metals present such as arsenic, lead, mercury, or cadmium. They should also be screened for contaminants such as other pharmaceuticals and be analyzed for pesticides, fungicides, insecticides, and other toxic ingredients.[4]

Many forms of nutrients are hardly bioavailable and they pass through your gut without being absorbed. For example, magnesium oxide is only one-tenth as bioavailable as magnesium aspartate.[5] However, manufactures will frequently use the oxide form because the aspartate form is more expensive and takes up a lot of room in the capsule.

Every year over 75 percent of your body is replaced and reconstructed from the nutrients you eat and take, even the DNA of your genes. The quality of these vitamins and nutrients determines the quality of your cells, how well they function, and prevent disease.

The dosages discussed in all the following sections of the book are for adults and are daily amounts. All dosages are in milligrams (mg) unless otherwise stated. If milligrams are not used the units of dosage are spelled out to avoid confusion. 1,000 micrograms equal one mg and 1,000 mg equal one gram.

Vitamin A

1

Vitamin A is a fat soluble vitamin. It is divided into two groups: aldehydes and carotenoids.
- Aldehydes: retinal, retinoic acid
- Carotenoids: beta-carotene, alpha-carotene, gama-carotene
  Beta-carotene is converted into vitamin A inside your gut.

Functions of vitamin A in your body:[1, 2, 3]
- Needed for the growth and support of the skin
- Required for vision
- Responsible for healthy mucous membranes
- Needed to detoxify PCBs and dioxin
- Immune function (improves white blood cells, natural killer cells, macrophages and T and B lymphocytes)
- Bone development
- Reduces your risk for cancer (esophageal, bladder, stomach, skin, leukemia, lymphoma)

Symptoms of vitamin A deficiency:[4, 5, 6]
- Night blindness
- Rough, scaly skin
- Fatigue
- Increased susceptibility to infections
- Poor wound healing
- Dry eyes

- Decreased steroid synthesis
- Increased vaginal yeast infections
- Hypothyroidism (low thyroid)
- Poor tooth and bone function

Causes of low vitamin A:[7, 8]
- Decreased intake of vitamin containing foods
- Antibiotics
- Laxatives
- Cholesterol-lowering medications
- Diabetes

Increases levels of vitamin A in your body:[9]
- Birth control pills

The following are food sources of vitamin A from most to least: liver (lamb), liver (beef), liver (calf), peppers (red chili), dandelion greens, liver (chicken), carrots, apricots (dried), collard greens, kale, sweet potatoes, parsley, spinach, turnip greens, mustard greens, Swiss chard, beet greens, chives, butternut squash, watercress, mangos, peppers (sweet, red), hubbard squash, cantaloupe, butter, endive, apricots, broccoli spears, whitefish, green onions, romaine lettuce, papayas, nectarines, prunes, pumpkin, swordfish, cream (whipping), peaches, acorn squash, eggs, chicken, cherries (sour red), butterhead lettuce, asparagus, tomatoes, peppers (green chili), kidneys, green peas, elderberries, watermelon, rutabagas, Brussels sprouts, okra, yellow cornmeal, and yellow squash.[10]

Dosage: 5,000-10,000 IU

Symptoms of vitamin A toxicity:[11]
- Weight loss
- Appetite loss
- Dry skin
- Hair loss
- Fatigue
- Bone pain
- Headache
- Irritability
- Joint pain

Side effects: Excess vitamin A intake can cause liver damage and even death. If you are taking a high dose your doctor should measure your calcium and liver enzymes on a regular basis.[12] *If you have liver disease, are a smoker, exposed to asbestos, or are pregnant you should not use high doses of vitamin A.* Also, a recent study suggests that even 5,000 IU *of vitamin A per day for more than 20 years from dietary sources can increase hip fractures in women.*[13]

The Carotenoids

There are over 700 carotenoids on the earth, only 60 are found in food. The typical American diet only includes six of them: alpha carotene, beta carotene, cryptoxanthin, lutein, lycopene, and zeaxanthin. Alpha carotene, beta carotene, and cryptoxanthin are converted into vitamin A by your body.

Lycopene
Functions in your body:[14, 15]
- Decreases LDL (bad) cholesterol
- Helps prevent prostate cancer
- Lowers blood pressure

Foods that contain lycopene:
- Tomatoes
- Watermelon
- Guavas
- Dark green leafy vegetables
- Pink grapefruit

Lycopene is best absorbed when cooked with fat such as the oil and cheese in pizza. *Fresh tomatoes are therefore not a good source of lycopene.* Lycopene is also present in guava, pink grapefruit, and watermelon.

Dosage: 5-20 mg

Lutein/Zeaxanthin
Functions of lutein and zeaxanthin in your body:
- Helps prevent cataracts and macular degeneration

Foods that contain lutein and zeaxanthin:
- Kale
- Collard greens
- Spinach
- Green leafy vegetables

Dosage: 6-12 mg

Cryptoxanthin

Cryptoxanthin is a carotenoid found in papayas, peaches, and oranges which may protect women against cervical cancer.

Side effects: Carotenoids have to be taken carefully. Pharmacologic doses of a single carotenoid may result in inhibiting the other carotenoids at the cellular level.[16]

Vitamin D

2

Vitamin D is a fat soluble vitamin. It is not really a vitamin but is actually a hormone. It is present in sunlight and your body absorbs vitamin D from the sun into your skin. The active form of vitamin D is called 1,25 dihydroxycholecalciferol. You can also get vitamin D in smaller doses from food. Vitamin D3 comes from red meat and fish. Vitamin D2 comes from plants. Boron may be needed to convert vitamin D to its active form. Your body has vitamin D receptors in your bones, pancreas, intestine, kidneys, brain, spinal cord, male and female reproductive organs, thymus, adrenal glands, pituitary, and thyroid gland.

Functions of vitamin D in your body:[1, 2, 3]
- Aids in the absorption of calcium from the intestinal tract
- Helps the body assimilate phosphorus
- Stimulates bone cell mineralization
- Helps the pancreas release insulin

Things that decrease vitamin D in your body:[4, 5]
- Aging (your body makes less vitamin D from the sun)
- Medications (e.g., phenytoin)
- Decreased fat absorption (short bowel syndrome, sprue, or medication that decreases fat absorption)
- Use of sunscreen (prevents vitamin D absorption)
- Prednisone interferes with the conversion of vitamin D to its active form

The following are food sources of vitamin D from most to least: sardines (canned), salmon, tuna, shrimp, butter, sunflower seeds, liver, eggs, milk (fortified), mushrooms, and natural cheese.[6]

Dosage:
- Adults under age 60: 400 IU
- Age 60-70: 600 IU
- Age 70 and above: 800 IU

Side effects: Doses of vitamin D greater than 1,200 IU should be avoided since your body stores vitamin D you may become toxic.

3

Vitamin E

Vitamin E is a group of compounds that consist of eight components:

- 4 are tocopherols: alpha, beta, gamma, and delta
- 4 are tocotrienols: alpha, beta, gamma, and delta

Alpha tocopherol is the most biologically active.

Functions of vitamin E in your body:[1, 2, 3, 4, 5, 6, 7]

- Antioxidant
- Can stop cholesterol-like substances from damaging your blood vessels and causing heart disease and stroke
- Can increase your immune system
- Ovaries need vitamin E to function properly
- Inhibits platelet adhesion
- Helps protect neurons in your brain from beta amyloid protein-induced oxidant toxicity (helps prevent Alzheimer's disease)
- Protects vitamin A and increases its storage
- Can act as an estrogen substitute and relieve hot flashes
- Helps relieve atrophic vaginitis
- Improves the action of insulin

Things that can decrease vitamin E levels:[8]
- High levels of vitamin A
- High intake of wheat bran
- High intake of pectin
- High intake of alcohol
- Smoking

The following are food sources of vitamin E from most to least: wheat germ, sunflower seeds, sunflower seed oil, safflower oil, almonds, sesame oil, peanut oil, corn oil, wheat germ, peanuts, olive oil, soybean oil, peanuts (roasted), peanut butter, butter, spinach, oatmeal, bran, asparagus, salmon, brown rice, rye (whole), dark rye bread, pecans, wheat germ, rye and wheat crackers, whole wheat bread, carrots, peas, walnuts, bananas, eggs, tomatoes, and lamb.[9]

Vitamin E is used to treat:[10, 11, 12]
- Prevent and treat heart disease
- Claudication (pain in legs with exercise)
- Fibrocystic breast disease
- PMS
- Hot flashes
- Painful menstrual cycles
- Hepatitis
- Restless leg syndrome
- Scleroderma/autoimmune diseases
- Osteoporosis

Side effects: Ferrous sulfate (iron) destroys vitamin E and therefore should not be taken with it. Other forms of iron, such as ferrous gluconate or ferrous fumarate leave vitamin E alone.[13] *If you are taking an anticoagulant (blood thinner) then use vitamin E with caution since it is also a blood thinner. Consequently, consult your physician if taking a blood thinner as to the amount of vitamin E that is right for you.* No toxicity is seen up to 3,200 IU.

Dosage: 100 to 1,200 IU. Vitamin E is recycled by vitamin C, alpha lipoic acid, and coenzyme Q-10. Vitamin E comes in natural and synthetic forms. Natural vitamin E is d-alpha (or d-beta, d-gamma, or d-delta) and synthetic vitamin E is noted as dl-alpha (or dl-beta, dl-gamma, or dl-delta). Natural vitamin E is better absorbed by your body and your liver does a better job of metabolizing it.[14]

Functions of tocotrienols alone:[15, 16, 17]
- Lower cholesterol
- Reverse plaque build-up
- Fight inflammation
- Reduce risk of cancer

Dosage: mixed tocotrienols, 100-300 mg. They should be taken with other antioxidants since they have a synergistic affect (work together). In our office we use Ultratrienols made by Designs for Health (see Appendix for availability).

Vitamin K

4

Vitamin K is a fat soluble vitamin that is made in your intestinal tract by friendly bacteria. It is also found in plants and synthesized by bacteria found in animal foods.

Functions of vitamin K in your body:[1, 2, 3]
- Helps your blood clot
- Is needed for the synthesis of osteocalcin for bone building
- Stimulates new bone growth
- Decreases the loss of calcium

Deficiency of vitamin K can cause:[4, 5, 6, 7]
- Increased breakdown of skin collagen
- Decrease in the amount of collagen in your skin which makes it look thinner
- Associated with an increase risk of coronary artery calcification
- Associated with a drop in vitamin C levels

Deficiency of vitamin K is due to:[8, 9, 10]
- Decrease in green leafy vegetables
- Cholesterol lowering drugs
- Antibiotic use (kills potassium making bacteria in the gut)
- Synthetic estrogen use

- Gallstones
- Liver disease
- Unhealthy intestinal tract
- Excess intake of vitamins A and E

If you are on an anticoagulant such as coumadin, you should eat less of the following foods that contain vitamin K (from most to least): turnip greens, broccoli, lettuce, cabbage, liver (beef), spinach, watercress, asparagus, cheese, butter, liver (pork), oats, green peas, whole wheat, green beans, pork, eggs, corn oil, peaches, beef, liver (chicken), raisins, tomato, milk, and potato.[11]

Side effects: The synthetic form may cause toxicity.

Dosage: 100 to 500 micrograms

5

The B Vitamins

It is important to have an adequate intake of all your B vitamins. The entire complex works together to help provide you with optimal health. B vitamins are water soluble and therefore should be taken at least twice a day since they are quickly eliminated from your body. If you are on estrogen replacement therapy or birth control pills, you should take extra B vitamins since hormonal therapy leads to a deficiency. Also, high dose supplementation of a single B vitamin can cause imbalances of other B vitamins. Therefore you should take B complex vitamins and not one B vitamin by itself.[1]

The following are your B vitamins:
- Thiamine (vitamin B1)
- Riboflavin (vitamin B2)
- Niacin (vitamin B3)
- Biotin
- Pantothenic acid (vitamin B5)
- Pyridoxine (vitamin B6)
- Para-aminobenzoic acid
- Choline
- Inositol
- Cyanocobalamin (vitamin B12)
- Folic acid

B vitamins perform the following functions in your body:[2]
- Glucose metabolism
- Inactivation of estrogen by the liver
- Stabilization of brain chemistry
- Used in thyroid function
- Helps relieve leg cramps

Symptoms of low B vitamins:[3]
- Insomnia
- Irritability
- Sugar cravings
- A change in appetite
- Impaired metabolism of medications
- Reduced immune system
- Poor scores in personality testing

1.1 Thiamine (B1)

Functions of thiamine in your body:[1, 2]
- Needed for proper metabolism of thyroid hormones
- Required for proper nerve function
- Used for activation of enzymes in the adrenal glands
- Needed for synthesis of nucleic acids and NADPH
- Used in the synthesis of acetylcholine
- Needed for energy production (Kreb cycle)
- Helps the body adapt to stress and avoid adrenal burnout
- Is needed for the making of aldosterone

Symptoms of thiamine deficiency:[3]
- Vision problems
- Irritability
- Confusion
- Poor memory
- Sleep disturbance
- Fatigue
- Forgetfulness
- Mild depression
- Gastrointestinal (gut) disturbances
- Loss of appetite
- Nervousness
- General weakness
- Headache
- Heart racing

Substances that decrease thiamine:[4, 5]

- Sugar
- Blueberries
- Red beet root
- Brussels sprouts
- Tea
- Antibiotics
- Sulfa drugs
- Oral contraceptives
- Alcohol (If you marinate your meat in wine, soy sauce or vinegar, it depletes the levels of thiamine by 50 to 75 percent.)
- Sulfites (a food additive)
- Diuretics (water pills)

The following are food sources of thiamine from most to least: yeast (brewer's), wheat germ, sunflower seeds, rice polishings, pine nuts, peanuts (with skins), Brazil nuts, pork, pecans, soybean flour, beans (pinto and red), split peas, millet, wheat bran, pistachio nuts, navy beans, buckwheat, oatmeal, whole-wheat flour, whole-wheat grain, lima beans (dry), hazelnuts, heart (lamb), wild rice, rye (whole-grain), cashews, liver (lamb), mung beans, cornmeal (whole-ground), lentils, kidneys (beef), green peas, macadamia nuts, brown rice, walnuts, garbanzo beans, garlic (cloves), liver (beef), almonds, lima beans (fresh), pumpkin and squash seeds, chestnuts (fresh), soybean sprouts, peppers (red chili), and sesame seeds (hulled).[6]

Grains lose up to 100 percent of their thiamine content when processed.[7]

Thiamine is used to treat:[8]

- Dementia
- Neuropathy
- Fatigue
- Alcoholism
- Confusion
- Depression
- Pain
- Memory loss

Side effects: High doses of thiamine may deplete your body of vitamin B6 or magnesium.[9]

Dosage: 10-100 mg

1.2 Riboflavin (B2)

Functions of riboflavin in your body:[1, 2]

- Needed for energy metabolism
- Needed to convert B6, folic acid, vitamin A, and niacin into its active form
- Required for proper thyroid function
- Used for the formation of aldosterone by the adrenal glands
- Used in lipid metabolism
- Involved in the metabolism of vitamin K
- Used in the cytochrome P450 system to metabolize medications and xenobiotics (environmental toxins) in your liver
- Needed in the regeneration of glutathione (the strongest antioxidant produced by your body)
- Is the catalyst in several reactions involved in the processing of carbohydrates fats, and proteins

Symptoms of riboflavin deficiency:

- Dry, cracking skin

Substances that reduce the bioavailability of riboflavin:[3, 4]

- Copper
- Zinc
- Caffeine
- Theophylline
- Saccharin
- Vitamin B3
- Vitamin C
- Tryptophan
- Alcohol
- Antacids
- Adriamycin
- Phenothiazines
- Phenytoin
- Imipramine
- Amitriptyline

The following are food sources of riboflavin from most to least: yeast (brewer's), liver (lamb), liver (beef), liver (calf), kidneys (beef), liver (chicken), kidneys (lamb), chicken (giblets), heart (veal), almonds, heart (beef), heart (lamb), wheat germ, wild rice, mushrooms, egg yolks, millet, peppers (hot red), soy flour, wheat bran, mackerel, collards, soybeans (dry), eggs, split peas, tongue (beef), kale, parsley, cashews, rice bran, veal, salmon, broccoli, pine nuts, sunflower seeds, pork, navy beans, beet and mustard greens, lentils, prunes, rye, whole grain, mung beans, beans (pinto and red), blackeyed peas, and okra.[5]

The processing of food decreases the riboflavin content by up to 80 percent.[6]

Riboflavin is used to treat:[7, 8]

- Acne
- Alcoholism
- Skin changes around the mouth
- Arthritis
- Athlete's foot
- Baldness
- Cataracts
- Depression
- Diabetes mellitus
- Diarrhea
- Visual changes
- Hysteria
- Indigestion
- Light sensitivity
- Nerve damage
- Reddening of eyes
- Scrotal skin changes
- Seborrhic dermatitis
- Stress
- Failure to detoxify effectively
- Migraines

Side effects: None.

Dosage: 10-100 mg. During illness and athletic training you need more riboflavin.

1.3 Niacin (B3)

Niacin is made from tryptophan, B6, B2, and iron. It is used in at least 40 chemical reactions in your system.

Functions of niacin in your body:[1, 2, 3]

- Needed for the proper function of the adrenal glands
- Is an element in two enzyme cofactors, NADH and NADPH which are involved in energy production
- Provides energy needed to convert cholesterol to pregnenolone (one of your sex hormones)
- Is used in the metabolism of carbohydrates, proteins, and fats
- Can lower LDL (bad) cholesterol and raise HDL (good) cholesterol
- May improve diabetes
- Decreased lipoprotein A (risk factor for heart disease)
- Lowers triglycerides
- Decreases fibrinogen (risk factor for heart disease)
- Used in the metabolism of tryptophan and serotonin

Symptoms of niacin deficiency:[4]

- Anorexia
- Nausea
- Skin changes around the mouth
- Confusion
- Depression
- Dermatitis
- Fatigue
- Mouth ulcers
- Headaches
- Indigestion
- Insomnia
- Irritability
- Muscle weakness
- Inability to detoxify

The following are food sources of niacin from most to least: yeast (brewer's), rice bran, rice polishings, wheat bran, peanuts (with skin), liver (lamb), liver (pork), peanuts (without skin), liver (beef), liver (calf), turkey (light meat), liver (chicken), chicken (light meat), trout, halibut, mackerel, heart (veal), chicken (fresh only), swordfish, turkey (fresh only), goose (fresh only), heart (beef), salmon, veal, kidneys (beef), wild rice, chicken giblets, lamb, chicken (flesh and skin), sesame seeds, sunflower seeds, beef, pork, brown rice, pine nuts, buckwheat (whole-grain), peppers (red chili), whole wheat grain, whole wheat flour, wheat germ, barley, herring, almonds, shrimp, split peas, and haddock.[5]

Side effects: High doses of niacin or extended release niacin should only be taken under the supervision of your doctor since liver damage, peptic ulcer, or decreased glucose metabolism can occur.[6] *Do not take niacin alone since it can elevate your homocysteine levels in your body. This increases your risk of heart disease and memory loss.[7] If statin drugs (cholesterol lowering) and niacin are used together rhabdomyolysis may occur.[8]*

Dosage: 50 mg-3,000 mg (see your doctor for use of doses greater than 100 mg).

Niacin is used to treat:[9, 10]

- Rheumatoid arthritis
- Osteoarthritis
- Diabetes mellitus
- Memory loss
- Intermittent claudication (pain in legs due to circulation changes)
- Depression
- High cholesterol
- High triglycerides
- Increases HDL
- Acne
- Parkinson's disease
- Painful menstrual cycles

1.4 Pantothenic Acid (B5)

Functions of pantothenic acid in your body:[1]

- Production of adrenal hormones
- Aids in the formation of antibodies
- Helps your body use other vitamins
- Helps convert food into energy
- Helps in antibody formation
- Aids in wound healing
- Needed for synthesis of coenzyme A part of the Krebs cycle (energy producing)

- Used in the synthesis of several amino acids
- Used to make vitamin D
- Needed to make fatty acids
- Used in red cell production
- Helps with fatty acid transport

Symptoms of pantothenic acid deficiency:[2, 3, 4]

- High blood pressure
- Depression
- Fatigue
- Headache
- Insomnia
- Burning sensation in your feet
- Enlarged, beefy, furrowed tongue
- Eczema
- Duodenal ulcers
- Intestinal inflammation
- Nerve degeneration
- Graying hair
- Gout
- Decreased antibody formation
- Upper respiratory tract infections
- Vomiting
- Restlessness
- Muscle cramps
- Constipation
- Adrenal exhaustion
- Allergies
- Arthritis
- Decreased production of hydrochloric acid in your stomach

Deficiency due to:[5]

- Sleeping pills
- Caffeine
- Estrogen supplementation

The following are food sources of pantothenic acid from most to least: yeast (brewer's), liver (calf), liver (chicken), kidneys (beef), peanuts, heart, mushrooms, soybean flour, split peas, tongue (beef), perch, blue cheese, pecans, soybeans, eggs, lobster, oatmeal (dry), buckwheat flour, sunflower seeds, lentils, rye flour (whole), cashews, salmon (fresh), Camembert cheese, garbanzos beans, wheat germ (toasted), broccoli, hazelnuts, turkey (dark meat), brown rice, whole-wheat flour, sardines, peppers (red chili), avocados, veal, black-eyed peas (dry), wild rice, cauliflower, chicken (dark meat), and kale.[6]

Dosage: 50 to 250 mg

Side effects: None.

Pantothenic acid is used to treat:[7, 8]

- Acne
- Osteoarthritis
- Rheumatoid arthritis
- Shingles
- Genital herpes and cold sores
- Ulcerative colitis

- Fatigue
- Infection
- Adrenal dysfunction
- Allergies
- Elevated triglycerides
- Problems with detoxification

1.5 Pyridoxine (B6)

Pyrodoxine acts as a partner for more than 100 different enzymes. The efficiency with which you utilize B6 declines with age.

Functions of pyridoxine in your body:[1]

- Used in methylation process (lowers homocysteine, a risk factor for heart disease and memory loss)
- Needed for the production of hydrocholoric acid
- Needed for the absorption of fats and proteins
- Key to the synthesis of several neurotransmitters including the metabolism of tryptophan to serotonin
- Needed for transfer of amino groups
- Used in the metabolism of amino acids
- Needed for the immune system
- Is a cofactor for an enzyme that strengthens connective tissue.
- Needed for REM sleep
- Detoxifies chemicals

Symptoms of pyridoxine deficiency:[2, 3]

- Fatigue
- Insomnia
- Skin lesions around the mouth
- Mouth ulcers
- Mental confusion
- Nervousness
- Weakness
- Irritability
- Hyperactivity
- Depression
- Numbness

Causes of pyridoxine deficiency:[4, 5, 6, 7, 8]

- Antidepressants
- Oral contraceptives
- Estrogen supplementation
- Cortisone
- Isonazid
- Dopamine
- Amphetamines
- Cigarette smoking
- Food additives (FDC yellow #5)
- Phenelzine
- Hydralazine
- Theophylline
- Pesticides
- Excessive exercise
- Aminoglycosides
- Chlortetracyline
- Doxycycline
- Fluroquinolones
- Hydrochlorothiazide
- Minocycline
- Penicillamine
- Raloxifene
- Theophilline
- Bumetanide
- Demeclocycline
- Penicillins
- Sulfonamides
- Torsemide
- Cephalosporins
- Diethylstylbesterol
- Ethancrynic acid
- Hydralazine
- Macrolides
- Oxytetracyline
- Quinestrol
- Tetracyclines
- Trimethoprim

The following are food sources of pyridoxine from most to least: yeast (brewer's), sunflower seeds, wheat germ (toasted), tuna (flesh), liver (beef), soybeans (dry), liver (chicken), walnuts, salmon (fresh), trout (fresh), liver (calf), mackerel (fresh), liver (pork), soybean flour, lentils (dry), lima beans (dry), buckwheat flour, black-eyed peas (dry), navy beans (dry), brown rice, hazelnuts, garbanzos (dry), pinto beans (dry), bananas, pork, albacore (fresh), halibut (fresh), kidneys (beef), avocados, kidneys (veal), whole-wheat flour, chestnuts (fresh), egg yolks, kale, rye flour, spinach, turnip greens, peppers (sweet), heart (beef), potatoes, prunes, raisins, sardines, Brussels sprouts, elderberries, perch (fresh), cod (fresh), barley, Camembert cheese, sweet potatoes, cauliflower, popcorn (popped), red cabbage, and leeks.[9]

Side effects: Pyridoxine can cause a neuropathy at too high a dose (more than 500 mg a day). *If you are taking L-dopa for Parkinson's disease you should not take B6 without the advice of your doctor.*[10, 11]

Dosage: 30 to 500 mg

Pyridoxine is used to treat:[12, 13]

- Asthma
- Carpal tunnel syndrome
- Epilepsy
- MSG sensitivity
- PMS
- Nausea and vomiting that occur with pregnancy
- Depression
- Atherosclerosis
- Osteoporosis
- Autism
- Irritability
- Eczema
- Diabetes mellitus
- Nervous system dysfunction
- Prevention of calcium oxalate kidney stones
- Seborrheic dermatitis
- Schizophrenia
- MSG intolerance
- Sickle cell disease
- Infertility

1.6 Cobalamin (B12)

Vitamin B12 is synthesized by bacteria. It exists in every animal food. Your body needs intrinsic factor secreted by your stomach and hydrocholoric acid in your stomach to absorb B12. Calcium is also needed for this process.[1]

Functions of B12 in your body:[2]
- Needed for red blood cell metabolism
- Needed for nervous system function
- Facilitates the metabolism of folic acid
- Functions as a methyl donor (lowers homocysteine, a risk factor for heart disease and memory loss)
- Involved in the production of neurotransmitters
- DNA synthesis
- Needed for carnitine metabolism

Symptoms of B12 deficiency:[3, 4, 5, 6]
- Decreased progesterone in women
- Decreased estrogen in women
- Increased cortisol levels
- Elevated levels of homocysteine
- Insomnia
- Memory loss
- Weakness
- Dizziness
- Sore tongue
- Confusion
- Fatigue
- Irritability
- Depression
- Moodiness
- Numbness and tingling in the extremities
- Drowsiness
- Stiffness
- Diarrhea
- Poor appetite

Substances that decrease B12 absorption:[7, 8]
- Potassium citrate and chloride
- Colchicine
- Some oral hypoglycemic agents (lower blood sugar)
- Antacids may decrease absorption from food but not supplementation

Drugs that deplete vitamin B12 from your body:[9]
- Aminoglycosides
- Cephalosporins
- Chlortetracyline
- Cholestyramine
- Cimetidine
- Co-trimoxazole
- Doxycycline
- Famotidine

- Fluroquinolones
- Lansoprazole
- Macrolides
- Metformin
- Minocycline
- Neomycin
- Nizatidine
- Omperazol
- Oral contraceptives
- Oxytetracycline
- Penicillins
- Phenytoin
- Rantidine
- Sulfonamides
- Tetracylines
- Trimethoprim

The following are food sources of cobalamin (B12) from most to least: liver (lamb), clams, liver (beef), kidneys (lamb), liver (calf), kidneys (beef), liver (chicken), oysters, sardines, heart (beef), egg yolks, heart (lamb), trout, salmon (fresh), tuna (fresh), lamb, sweetbreads (thymus), eggs, whey (dried), beef, Edam cheese, Swiss cheese, brie cheese, Gruyere cheese, blue cheese, haddock (fresh), flounder (fresh), scallops, cheddar cheese, cottage cheese, mozzarella cheese, halibut, perch (fillets), and swordfish (fresh).[10]

Side effects: None.

Dosage: 400 to 5,000 micrograms

B12 is used in the treatment of the following conditions:[11, 12, 13]

- Anemia
- Asthma
- Fatigue
- Hepatitis
- Dementia
- Epilepsy
- Depression
- Psychosis
- Irritability
- Ataxia
- Numbness
- Tingling
- Neuropathy
- AIDS
- Multiple sclerosis
- Tinnitus
- Infertility
- Anxiety
- Insomnia
- Retinopathy
- Sciatica
- Trigeminal neuralgia
- Bell's palsy
- Leg cramps (night)
- Vitiligo
- Xanthelasmia
- Seborrheic dermatitis

1.7 Biotin

Biotin is a B vitamin. The flora of your gastrointestinal tract (gut) makes biotin. If you take antibiotics all of the time, the bacteria that synthesizes biotin are killed off and you will not make enough.

Functions of biotin in your body:[1, 2]

- Strengthens nails
- Used in energy metabolism
- Needed for fatty acid synthesis
- Increases insulin sensitivity

Deficiency of biotin can cause:[3]

- Hair loss
- Scaly dermatitis
- Nausea
- Depression
- Hallucinations
- Reduced appetite
- Muscle pain
- Localized numbness and tingling
- Cradle cap in the newborn
- Dandruff

Things that cause a deficiency of biotin:[4, 5, 6]

- Alcohol excess
- Raw egg whites
- Anticonvulsants (phenytoin, carbamazepine, primidone, phenobarbital)

What increases biotin:

- Vegetarian diet

The following are food sources of biotin from most to least: brewer's yeast, liver (lamb), liver (pork), liver (beef), soy flour, soybeans, rice bran, rice germ, rice polishings, egg yolk, peanut butter, walnuts, peanuts (roasted), barley, pecans, oatmeal, sardines (canned), whole egg, black-eyed peas, split peas, almonds, cauliflower, mushrooms, whole-wheat cereal, salmon (canned), textured vegetable protein, bran, lentils, and brown rice.[7]

Side effects: None.

Dosage: 300 to 600 micrograms. Doses of up to 3,000 micrograms have been used under the supervision of a physician.

Biotin is used to treat the following conditions:[8, 9, 10, 11]
- Seborrheic dermatitis
- Diabetes mellitus
- Diabetic neuropathy
- Brittle nails

1.8 Inositol

Inositol is part of the vitamin B complex.

Functions of inositol in your body:[1]
- Involved in augmenting effects of neurotransmitter release
- Calming affect
- Helps increase sleep quality
- Involved with how the liver handles fat
- Supports the metabolism of estrogen and progesterone

Signs of inositol deficiency:[2]
- Difficulty falling asleep
- PMS symptoms
- Fibroid tumors
- Depression
- Anxiety

Foods that contain inositol include fruits, beans, grains, and nuts.[3]

Dosage: 200 milligrams to 12 grams (dosages larger than 200 micrograms need physician supervision).

Side effects: If you have kidney failure you should not take inositol.

Inositol is used to treat:[4, 5, 6, 7]
- Panic attacks
- Neuropathy
- PMS
- Fibroids
- Liver support
- Depression

1.9 Folic acid

Folate is the name given to a group of compounds that share a common molecular architecture. It is also called folic acid and folacin. Part of the folic acid you need is made in the intestine.

Functions of folic acid in your body:[1, 2, 3]

- Needed for proper health of all tissues especially mucous membrane tissues of the digestive tract, vagina, and cervix
- Protects baby from neural tube defects such as spina bifida
- Involved in methylation (decreases homocysteine)
- Produces S-adenosylmethionine (SAMe)
- Metabolic conversion of dopamines
- Detoxifies hormones (estrogen)
- Produces complex phospholipids for neurological function (COMT)
- Detoxifies phenols from the environment
- Needed for the synthesis of hemoglobin
- DNA metabolism
- Central nervous system function

Folic acid deficiency is associated with:[4, 5, 6, 7, 8, 9]

- Increased risk of cervical cancer
- Increased risk of heart disease and memory loss due to high homocysteine levels
- Increased number of ovarian cysts
- Impaired synthesis of estrogen and progesterone by the ovaries
- Low vitamin C levels
- Adrenal dysfunction
- Depression
- Anemia

Substances that cause a deficiency of folic acid:[10, 11, 12]

- Trimethoprim
- Triamterene
- Carbamazepine
- Phenytoin
- Phenobarbital
- Primidone
- Tobacco
- Alcohol
- Birth control pills
- Sulfasalazine
- Aspirin
- Celecoxib
- Colestipol
- Famotidine
- Indomethacin
- NSAIDs
- Barbituates
- Cholestyramine
- Corticosteroids
- Fosphentoin
- Methotrexate
- Ranitidine
- Cimetidine
- Ethosuximide
- Hydroclorothiazide
- Methsuxemide
- Salsalate
- Valproic acid

Symptoms of folic acid deficiency:[13]

- Weakness
- Inflamed and sore tongue that appears smooth and shiny
- Numbness or tingling in hands ands and feet
- Indigestion
- Diarrhea
- Depression
- Irritability
- Drowsiness
- Slow, weakened pulse
- Graying hair
- Mental illness
- Impaired wound healing
- Decreased resistance to infection
- Birth defects (neural tube)
- Toxemia
- Insomnia

The following are food sources of folic acid from most to least: brewer's yeast, black-eyed peas, rice germ, soy flour, wheat germ, liver (beef), liver (lamb), soy beans, liver (pork), bran, kidney beans, mung beans, lima beans, navy beans, garbanzo beans, asparagus, lentils, walnuts, spinach (fresh), kale, filbert nuts, beet and mustard greens, textured vegetable protein, peanuts (roasted), peanut butter, broccoli, barley, split peas, whole-wheat cereal, Brussels sprouts, almonds, whole-wheat flour, oatmeal, cabbage, dried figs, avocado, green beans, corn, coconut (fresh), pecans, mushrooms, dates, blackberries, ground beef, and oranges.[14]

Side effects: Dosages should not exceed 400 micrograms per day since folic acid supplementation may mask the symptoms of B12 deficiency. Large doses can cause insomnia, irritability, and gastrointestinal problems.[15] If you are taking phenytoin do not take high doses of folic acid.

Dosage: up to 400 micrograms a day. Higher doses may be used under the direction of a physician.

Folic acid is used to treat:[16]

- Cervical dysplasia
- Prevent birth defects (neural tube and cleft palate)
- Lower homocysteine
- Gout
- Restless leg syndrome
- Gingivitis
- Depression
- Psoriasis
- Cancer prevention

Vitamin C

6

Vitamin C cannot be made by humans, it must be taken in.

Functions of vitamin C in your body:[1, 2, 3, 4, 5, 6, 7, 8, 9, 10, 11]

- Is an antioxidant
- Prevents formation of nitrosamines
- Benefits immune system by increasing: white blood cells, interferon (proteins that fight viruses, production of lymphocytes)
- Prevents incidence of lung disease
- Decreases rate of stomach cancer
- Increases fertility
- Decreases rate of gum disease
- Lowers the incidence of cataracts
- Reduces bruising
- Aids in wound healing
- Helps regenerate vitamin E, glutathione, uric acid
- Involved in catecholamine synthesis
- Prevents free radical damage of LDL (bad) cholesterol
- Aids in the synthesis of collagen
- Helps carnitine synthesis
- Decreases risk of heart disease
- Helps in the metabolism of tyrosine
- Needed for progesterone production
- Reserves the energy producing capacity of the mitochondria

- Needed to maintain good levels of glutathione
- Reduces damage due to glycation
- Lowers sorbitol levels to prevent cataracts
- Involved in serotonin production
- Lowers blood pressure
- Decreases leukotrienes
- Is a diuretic
- Increases nitric oxide
- Decreases adrenal steroid production
- Lowers triglycerides
- Increases HDL (good cholesterol)

Symptoms of vitamin C loss:[12]

- Fatigue
- Bleeding gums
- Impaired wound healing
- Joint pain
- Loose teeth
- Easy bruising
- Frequent infections
- Cardiovascular disease

Things that cause you to have a lower vitamin C level:[13, 14]

- Stress
- Aging
- Smoking
- Diabetes mellitus
- Birth control pills
- High blood pressure
- High fever
- Sulfa drugs
- Pain killers
- Antibiotics
- Cortisone
- Aspirin

The following are food sources of vitamin C from most to least: peppers (red chili), guavas, peppers (red sweet), kale leaves, parsley, collard leaves, turnip greens, peppers (green sweet), broccoli, Brussels sprouts, mustard greens, watercress, cauliflower, persimmons, cabbage (red), strawberries, papayas, spinach, oranges and juice, cabbage, lemon juice, grapefruit and juice, elderberries, liver (calf), turnips, mangos, asparagus, cantaloupes, Swiss chard, green onions, liver (beef), okra, tangerines, New Zealand spinach, oysters, lima beans (young), black-eyed peas, soybeans, green peas, radishes, raspberries, Chinese cabbage, yellow summer squash, loganberries, honeydew melon, and tomatoes.[15]

The vitamin C content of foods is easily destroyed by light, heat, and chemicals. Fresh cut lettuce loses half of its vitamin C in 48 hours unless stored in a dark refrigerator.[16]

Side effects: If you have hemochromatosis you may experience an increased amount of iron uptake if you intake vitamin C.[17] If you have glucose-6-phosphate dehydrogenase deficiency (G-6PD) you should not have vitamin C given to you intravenously.[18]

Dosage: 1,000 to 5,000 mg. Higher doses may be used but can cause diarrhea.

Buffered forms that cause less diarrhea are the following:

• Mineral ascorbates where vitamin C is buffered with trace minerals such as calcium, magnesium, or zinc.

• Ester-C

If you are diabetic you need to take vitamin C. Vitamin C and glucose are used in the same pathway by your cells. Consequently, vitamin C will be competing with glucose to enter your cells and glucose will win. This leaves your cells deficient in vitamin C.[19]

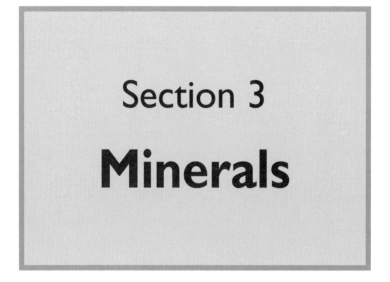

Section 3

Minerals

This section discusses the roles of different minerals by outlining each mineral's function, food sources, therapeutic uses, and side effects. Minerals are not produced by plants or animals.

Your body's biological function requires 18 different minerals. They serve many different functions. Minerals are divided into major and minor groups. Major minerals are present in your body in amounts greater than 5 grams. Minor minerals occur in amounts less than 5 grams.

Major Minerals

- Calcium
- Magnesium
- Phosphorus
- Sodium
- Chloride
- Potassium

Minor Minerals

- Arsenic
- Boron
- Chromium
- Cobalt
- Copper
- Fluoride
- Iodine
- Iron
- Manganese
- Molybdenum
- Nickel
- Selenium
- Silicon
- Tin
- Vanadium
- Zinc

Like vitamins and other nutrients, mineral intake is different based on your own individual dietary input, mineral content of the soil the food is grown in, medications taken, the function of your gut, and the interaction of other substances.

1

Calcium

Calcium is the most abundant mineral in your body.

Functions of calcium in your body:[1]
- Helps cholesterol make your sex hormones
- Responsible for bone and teeth development
- Muscles use calcium to aid in energy production
- Regulates ion transport in your cells
- Blood-clotting
- Activation of numerous enzymes
- Nerve impulse transmission
- Needed for the absorption of vitamin B12

Symptoms of calcium loss:
- Bone loss (osteoporosis)
- Muscle spasms and twitching
- Hypertension

Substances that increases calcium absorption:[2]
- Hydrochloric acid
- Ascorbic acid
- Citric acid
- Glycine
- Lysine

Substances that decrease calcium concentration in your body:[3, 4, 5, 6, 7, 8, 9, 10]

- Increased fat diet
- Fiber (supplementation should not be taken within two hours)
- Whole wheat
- Heavy exercise
- Chocolate
- Caffeine
- Alcohol
- Excess protein in your diet
- Sugar
- Aspartame
- Oxalic acid containing foods (spinach, kale, rhubarb, cocoa)
- High phosphorus containing foods (white flour, soft drinks)
- Increased zinc
- Steroids
- Tetracycline
- Excessive thyroid replacement
- Phenobarbital
- Heparin
- Methotrexate
- Cholestyramine
- Acidic foods (destroy your bones by stealing alkalizing minerals)

The following are acid creating foods:[11]

- Fruits: cranberry, blueberry, dried fruits
- Nuts and grains: oats, barley, rice, wheat, white bread, peanuts, walnuts, processed soybeans
- Vegetables: corn, processed
- Meats and dairy products: beef, veal, turkey, chicken, ham, haddock, milk, cheese, yogurt, ice cream, butter
- Drinks: coffee, beer, black tea, soft drinks
- Other: sugar, chocolate, honey, aspirin, white vinegar

Food Sources Of Calcium:

Mg per 100 grams edible portion (100 grams = 3 ½ oz.)

1093	Kelp	73	Soybeans, cooked
925	Swiss cheese	73	Pecans
750	Cheddar cheese	72	Wheat germ
352	Carob flour	69	Peanuts
296	Dulse	68	Miso
250	Collard leaves	68	Romaine lettuce
246	Turnip greens	67	Dried apricots
245	Barbados molasses	66	Rutabaga
234	Almonds	62	Raisins
210	Brewer's yeast	60	Black currant
203	Parsley	59	Dates
200	Corn tortillas (lime added)	56	Green snap beans
		51	Globe artichoke
187	Dandelion greens	51	Dried prunes
186	Brazil nuts	51	Pumpkin and squash seeds
151	Watercress		
129	Goat's milk	50	Cooked dry beans
128	Tofu	49	Common cabbage
126	Dried figs	48	Soybean sprouts
121	Buttermilk	46	Hard winter wheat
120	Yogurt	41	Orange
119	Beet greens	39	Celery
119	Wheat bran	38	Cashews
118	Whole milk	38	Rye grain
114	Buckwheat, raw	37	Carrot
110	Sesame seeds, hulled	34	Barley
106	Ripe olives	32	Sweet potato
103	Broccoli	32	Brown rice
99	English walnut	29	Garlic
94	Cottage cheese	28	Summer squash
93	Spinach	27	Onion

26	Lemon	16	Beets
26	Fresh green peas	14	Cantaloupe
25	Cauliflower	14	Jerusalem artichoke
25	Lentils, cooked	13	Tomato
22	Sweet cherry	12	Eggplant
22	Asparagus	12	Chicken
22	Winter squash	11	Orange juice
21	Strawberry	10	Beef
20	Millet	8	Banana
19	Mung bean sprouts	7	Apple
17	Pineapple	3	Sweet corn
16	Grapes		

Reprinted with permission from *Clinical Nutrition: A Functional Approach* by Jeffrey Bland.[12]

Side effects: Toxicity of calcium can occur due to several disease processes. Furthermore, if you intake too much calcium problems may occur.

Excess calcium supplementation can:[13, 14, 15]
- Clog your arteries (predispose you to heart disease)
- Block the uptake of manganese in your body
- Interfere with the absorption of magnesium
- Decrease iron absorption
- Interfere with the absorption of zinc
- Interfere with the making of vitamin K
- Cause kidney stones
- Cause your thyroid not to convert T4 to T3 (the more active form)

Dosage:
- Adults: 800 mg
- Pregnant or lactating women: 1,200 mg
- Peri-menopausal women: 1,000 mg
- Menopausal women: 1,600 mg

Your body can only absorb 500 mg of calcium at a time. Therefore, you should take it in divided doses. The above amounts are your daily intake between what you eat *and* what you take as a supplement.

Other important factors concerning calcium:[16, 17, 18, 19, 20]

- Milk is not the best source of calcium since pasteurization destroys up to 32% of the available calcium.
- Tums are not a good source of calcium intake. It is poorly absorbed.
- Always use only pharmaceutical grade supplements. Lower grade products may be contaminated with lead, mercury, arsenic, aluminum, and cadmium. (See Appendix for a list of pharmaceutical grade companies.)
- Vitamin C increases calcium absorption by 100%.
- Calcium carbonate is not the best form of calcium to use. Calcium citrate or hydroxyappetite are more bioavailable.

Calcium is used in the treatment or prevention of:[21]

- Osteoporosis
- Leg cramps
- Colon cancer
- Increased cholesterol
- Elevated triglycerides
- High blood pressure
- Preeclampsia
- PMS

Calcium interactions:[22]

- May interfere with the absorption of magnesium, zinc, iron, manganese, and phosphorus
- Inhibits absorption of tetracycline
- Decreases absorption of ciprofloxacin and most fluroquinolone antibiotics
- Increases the toxicity of digoxin
- Decreases aluminum absorption
- Interferes with the absorption of thyroid medication

Magnesium

2

Magnesium is involved in over 300 enzymes used in your body. It is a cofactor for the production of ATP, your energy source. One-half of the magnesium in your body is found in your bones.

Functions of magnesium in your body:[1, 2, 3, 4, 5, 6, 7, 8, 9, 10]

- Growth
- Pregnancy
- Sleep
- Wound healing
- Heart function
- Muscle relaxation
- Nerve function
- Skeletal muscle function
- Steroid hormone production
- Bone building
- Decreases blood vessel constriction
- Fatty acid synthesis and oxidation
- Protein synthesis
- Energy production
- Removes excess ammonia
- Improves glucose uptake by insulin
- Aids survival post bypass surgery

- Enhances the function of various brain antioxidants
- Prevents the production of chemicals in the body which increase inflammation
- Acts as a natural tranquilizer
- Is a natural anticonvulsant
- Maintains the normal rhythm of your heart
- Increases HDL (good cholesterol)
- Important in immune function
- Improves muscle strength and endurance
- Relaxes electrical impulses

Symptoms of magnesium loss:[11, 12]

- Muscle cramps
- Muscle twitches
- Back, neck pain/or spasm
- TMJ pain
- Muscle soreness
- Chest tightness
- Weakness
- Decreased appetite
- Irritability
- Fatigue
- Depression
- Anxiety
- Insomnia
- Hyperventilation
- Confusion
- Memory loss
- Chest tightness

Magnesium deficiency has been associated with the following:[13, 14, 15, 16, 17, 18, 19]

- Seizures
- Psychosis
- Delirium
- Tremors
- Heart attacks/cardiovascular disease
- Heart arrhythmia (irregular heart rate)
- PMS
- Osteoporosis
- Abnormal calcium deposits
- Poor wound healing
- Hypertension
- Difficulty swallowing
- Problem pregnancy
- Hypoglycemia
- Excitability
- Aggressive behavior
- Alcoholism
- Anxiety
- ADD (attention deficit disorder)

- Autism
- Dementia (memory loss)
- Depression
- Fatigue
- Insomnia
- Learning disabilities
- Schizophrenia
- Constipation
- Urinary spasm
- Photophobia
- Cold hands and feet
- Loud noise sensitivity
- Numbness
- Agoraphobia
- Tingling
- Mitral valve prolapse
- Palpitations
- Salt craving
- Carbohydrate craving
- Endometriosis
- Mental confusion
- Diabetes
- Lupus
- Migraine headaches
- Stress

Loss of magnesium can occur with:[20, 21]

- Diarrhea
- Trauma
- Surgery
- Extreme athletic competition
- Alcoholism
- Excessive sugar intake
- Fiber excess
- Caffeine intake
- Trans fatty acids
- Phosphates in soft drinks
- Stress
- Digoxin use
- Foods high in oxalic acid (almonds, cocoa, spinach, tea)
- Laxatives
- Asthma medications (beta-agonists, epinephrine)
- Diuretics (water pills), except potassium sparing
- Antibiotics (gentamicin, carbenicillin, amphotericin B)
- Drugs for chemotherapy (cis-platinum, vinblastine, bleomycin)
- Cyclosporine
- Steroids

Food Sources Of Magnesium:

MG per 100 grams edible portion (100 grams = 3 ½ oz.)

760	Kelp	38	Sunflower seeds
490	Wheat bran	37	Common beans, cooked
336	Wheat germ	37	Barley
270	Almonds	36	Dandelion greens
267	Cashews	36	Garlic
258	Blackstrap molasses	35	Raisins
231	Brewer's yeast	35	Fresh green peas
229	Buckwheat	34	Potato with skin
225	Brazil nut	34	Crab
220	Dulse	33	Banana
184	Filberts	31	Sweet potato
175	Peanuts	30	Blackberry
162	Millet	25	Beets
160	Wheat grain	24	Cauliflower
142	Pecan	23	Carrot
131	English walnut	22	Celery
115	Tofu	21	Beef
106	Beet greens	20	Asparagus
90	Coconut meat, dry	19	Chicken
88	Soybeans, cooked	18	Green pepper
88	Spinach	17	Winter squash
88	Brown rice	16	Cantaloupe
71	Dried figs	16	Eggplant
65	Swiss chard	14	Tomato
62	Apricots, dried	13	Cabbage
58	Dates	13	Grapes
57	Collard leaves	13	Milk
51	Shrimp	13	Mushroom
48	Sweet corn	12	Onion
45	Avocado	11	Orange
45	Cheddar cheese	11	Iceberg lettuce
41	Parsley	9	Plum
40	Prunes, dried	8	Apple

Reprinted with permission from *Clinical Nutrition: A Functional Approach* by Jeffrey Bland.[22]

Side effects: Diarrhea may occur if you have taken more than 600 mg of magnesium in a day. Symptoms of more severe toxicity include drowsiness, lethargy, and weakness.[23]

Dosage: 600-800 mg

Magnesium is used in the treatment of:[24]
- Chronic fatigue syndrome
- Fibromyalgia
- Mitral valve prolapse
- Heart attack
- Cardiac arrhythmias (irregular heart rhythm)
- Angina
- Congestive heart failure
- Cardiomyopathy (enlarged heart)
- Claudication (pain in legs due to decreased circulation)
- Low HDL (good cholesterol)
- Calcium-oxalate kidney stones
- Asthma
- Osteoporosis
- Migraine
- PMS
- Urinary symptoms
- Diabetes mellitus
- Hypoglycemia (low blood sugar)
- COPD (chronic obstructive pulmonary disease)
- Pregnancy
- High blood pressure
- Sickle cell disease
- Restless leg syndrome
- Spasms

Phosphorus

3

Most Americans are not deficient in phosphorus since phosphorus is contained in soft drinks and fast foods.

Functions of phosphorus in your body:[1]
- Component of bone and teeth
- Needed for energy production
- Helps regulate enzymes
- Part of the buffering system
- Is part of the structure of every cell in your body (part of nucleic acids)
- Repair and development of body tissue
- Lipid metabolism

Symptoms of low phosphorus:[2]
- Anorexia
- Weakness
- Fragile bones
- Joint stiffness

Can be deficient due to:
- Excess calcium intake
- Vitamin D deficiency
- Over consumption of antacids

Food Sources Of Phosphorus

Mg per 100 grams edible portion (100 grams = 3 ½ oz.)

1753	Brewer's yeast	119	Lentils, cooked
1276	Wheat bran	116	Mushrooms
1144	Pumpkin and squash seeds	116	Fresh peas
1118	Wheat germ	111	Sweet corn
837	Sunflower seeds	101	Raisins
693	Brazil nuts	93	Whole cow's milk
592	Sesame seeds, hulled	88	Globe artichoke
554	Soybeans, dried	87	Yogurt
504	Almonds	80	Brussels sprouts
478	Cheddar cheese	79	Prunes, dried
457	Pinto beans, dried	78	Broccoli
409	Peanuts	77	Figs, dried
400	Wheat	69	Yams
380	English walnut	67	Soybean sprouts
376	Rye grain	64	Mung bean sprouts
373	Cashews	63	Dates
353	Beef liver	63	Parsley
338	Scallops	62	Asparagus
311	Millet	59	Bamboo shoots
290	Barley, pearled	56	Cauliflower
289	Pecans	53	Potato with skin
267	Dulse	51	Okra
240	Kelp	51	Spinach
239	Chicken	44	Green beans
221	Brown rice	44	Pumpkin
205	Eggs	42	Avocado
202	Garlic	40	Beet greens
175	Crab	39	Swiss chard
152	Cottage cheese	38	Winter squash
150	Beef or lamb	36	Carrot
		36	Onions

35	Red cabbage	26	Lettuce
33	Beets	24	Nectarine
31	Radish	22	Raspberries
29	Summer squash	20	Grapes
28	Celery	20	Orange
27	Cucumber	17	Olives
27	Tomato	16	Cantaloupe
26	Banana	10	Apple
26	Persimmon	8	Pineapple
26	Eggplant		

Reprinted with permission form *Clinical Nutrition: A Functional Approach* by Jeffrey Bland.[3]

Side effects: No toxic levels have been reported.

Dosage:
- Adults ages 19-24: 2,400 mg
- Adults ages 25 and older: 800 mg
- Pregnant women: 1,200 mg

4

Potassium, Sodium, Chloride

Potassium, sodium, and choloride are minerals that are the electrolytes in your body. They are involved with the intracellular and extracellular fluid compartments of your cells. The major minerals in your extracellar compartments are sodium and chloride. The major component in the intacellular part is potassium. Maintaining a balance between the intra and extracellar compartments regulates many functions including nerve transmission and muscle contractions.

Sodium plays an important role in the transport of carbon dioxide, muscle contraction, nerve transmission, and amino acid transport.[1]

Food Sources Of Sodium:

Mg per 100 grams edible portion (100 grams = 3 ½ oz.)

3007	Kelp	229	Cottage cheese
2400	Green olives	210	Lobster
2132	Salt, 1 teaspoon	147	Swiss chard
1428	Dill pickles	130	Beet greens
1319	Soy sauce, 1 tablespoon	130	Buttermilk
828	Ripe olives	126	Celery
747	Sauerkraut	122	Eggs
700	Cheddar cheese	110	Cod
265	Scallops	71	Spinach

70	Lamb	27	Raisins
65	Pork	26	Red cabbage
64	Chicken	19	Garlic
60	Beef	19	White beans
60	Beets	15	Broccoli
60	Sesame seeds	15	Mushrooms
52	Watercress	13	Cauliflower
50	Whole cow's milk	10	Onion
49	Turnip	10	Sweet potato
47	Carrot	9	Lettuce
47	Yogurt	6	Cucumber
45	Parsley	5	Peanuts
43	Artichoke	4	Avocado
34	Dried figs	3	Tomato
30	Lentils, dried	2	Eggplant
30	Sunflower seeds		

Reprinted with permission from *Clinical Nutrition: A Functional Approach* by Jeffrey Bland.[2]

The remainder of this chapter discusses potassium.

Functions of potassium in your body:[3]

• Needed for muscle contraction
• Preserves the acid-base balance in your body
• Regulates fluid balance
• Needed for nerve transmission
• Used in glucose and glycogen metabolism
• Aids in maintaining cellular integrity

Symptoms of potassium loss:[4]

• Central nervous system changes
• Muscle weakness
• Slow heart rate
• Fragile bones
• Death

Things that cause a low potassium:[5]

- Diarrhea
- Vomiting
- Kidney disease
- Aging
- Starvation
- Burns
- Medications (diuretics/water pills)

Food Sources Of Potassium:

Mg per 100 grams edible portion (100 grams = 3 ½ oz.)

8060	Dulse	370	Meats
5273	Kelp	369	Winter squash
920	Sunflower seeds	366	Chicken
827	Wheat germ	341	Carrots
773	Almonds	341	Celery
763	Raisins	322	Radishes
727	Parsley	295	Cauliflower
715	Brazil nuts	282	Watercress
674	Peanuts	278	Asparagus
648	Dates	268	Red cabbage
640	Figs, dried	264	Lettuce
604	Avocado	251	Cantaloupe
603	Pecans	249	Lentils, cooked
600	Yams	244	Tomato
550	Swiss chard	243	Sweet potato
540	Soybeans, cooked	234	Papaya
529	Garlic	214	Eggplant
470	Spinach	213	Green pepper
450	English walnuts	208	Beets
430	Millet	202	Summer squash
416	Beans, cooked	200	Orange
414	Mushrooms	199	Raspberries
407	Potato with skin	191	Cherries
382	Broccoli	164	Strawberries
370	Banana	162	Grapefruit juice

158	Grapes	130	Pear
157	Onions	129	Eggs
146	Pineapple	110	Apple
144	Milk, whole	100	Watermelon
141	Lemon juice	70	Brown rice, cooked

Reprinted with permission from *Clinical Nutrition: A Functional Approach* by Jeffrey Bland.[6]

Side effects: *Potassium levels may need to be watched for toxicity if you are taking potassium-sparing medications such as aldactone or ACE inhibitors.*

Dosage: *500 mg. Magnesium deficiency will make potassium loss worse.*

Potassium is used in the treatment of:[7]
- High blood pressure
- Stroke prevention
- Diabetes mellitus
- Fatigue
- Postural low blood pressure

5

Boron

Boron is a minor or trace mineral.

Functions of boron in your body:[1, 2, 3, 4, 5, 6]
- Increases absorption of calcium, magnesium, and phosphorus
- Increases estrogen production in women
- Aids vitamin D to increase mineral content in your bone
- Enhances cartilage formation
- Increases the electrical activity of the brain
- Reduces prostate cancer risk
- Decreases inflammation
- Helps maintain memory

Food sources of boron:
- Apples
- Pears
- Peaches
- Grapes
- Nuts
- Legumes
- Cauliflower
- Broccoli
- Green leafy vegetables like kale

Side effects: usually seen in doses above 300 mg a day. They include nausea, vomiting, diarrhea, dermatitis, and lethargy.[7] More than 50 mg a day of boron can interfere with phosphorus and riboflavin metabolism.[8]

Dosage: 1,000 micrograms

6

Chromium

Chromium is not absorbed well into your body since it is molecularly a large mineral. It usually needs to be combined with another substance to allow it to enter the blood stream easily. Picolinate is a protein that serves this function well. Picolinate is found in living cells. It also increases the absorption of zinc, copper, and iron.

Functions of chromium in your body:[1, 2, 3, 4, 5, 6, 7, 8, 9]

- Helps decrease sugar cravings
- Burns calories
- Increases physical endurance in athletes
- Stimulates muscle development
- Reduces bone loss
- Helps raise DHEA levels
- Increases immunoglobulins
- Decreases cortisol
- Raises HDL (good cholesterol)
- Decreases total cholesterol and LDL (bad) cholesterol
- Helps hold onto calcium to prevent osteoporosis
- Aids in fat loss
- Helps regulate blood sugar by making insulin work more effectively

Signs of chromium deficiency:[10]
- Hyperglycemia/impaired glucose tolerance (high blood sugar)
- Increased cholesterol/triglycerides
- Neuropathy
- Elevated insulin
- Decreased insulin binding/receptor number
- Hypoglycemia (low blood sugar)

Causes of chromium loss:[11, 12]
- Antacid use
- High carbohydrate diet
- Exercise

Factors that increase chromium:[13, 14, 15]
- Amino acids
- Vitamin C
- Physical trauma

Food Sources Of Chromium:
Micrograms per 100 grams edible portion (100 grams = 3 ½ oz.)

112	Brewer's yeast	13	Butter
57	Beef, round	13	Parsnips
55	Calf's liver	12	Cornmeal
42	Whole wheat bread	12	Lamb chop
38	Wheat bran	11	Scallops
30	Rye bread	11	Swiss cheese
30	Fresh chili	10	Banana
26	Oysters	10	Spinach
24	Potatoes	10	Pork chop
23	Wheat germ	9	Carrots
19	Green pepper	8	Navy beans, dry
16	Eggs	7	Shrimp
15	Chicken	7	Lettuce
14	Apple	5	Orange

5	Lobster tail	4	Mushrooms
5	Blueberries	3	Beer
4	Green beans	3	Strawberries
4	Cabbage	1	Milk

Reprinted with permission from *Clinical Nutrition: A Functional Approach* by Jeffrey Bland.[16]

Side effects: lightheadedness, rash.

Dosage: 50-200 micrograms. Higher dosages may be used to treat a specific disease process. Up to 90% of the chromium content of food is lost in food processing.

7

Copper

The highest levels of copper in your body are found in the kidneys, liver, brain, and bone.

Functions of copper in your body:[1]
- Thyroid function (converts T4 to T3)
- Makes red blood cells
- White blood cells formation
- Connective tissue synthesis including collagen
- Antioxidant protection
- Skeletal mineralization
- Myelin formation
- Catecholamine metabolism
- Oxidative phosphorylation
- Cholesterol metabolism
- Immune function
- Heart function
- Glucose metabolic regulation
- Melanin pigment synthesis
- Protein metabolism
- Thermal regulation
- Needed for the production of adrenal and ovarian hormones
- Promotes healthy nerve function
- Helps wound healing
- Aids in energy production
- Decreases inflammation

Symptoms of copper deficiency:[2]
- Anemia (hypochromic microcytic)
- Low white count
- Decreased hair and skin pigmentation
- Failure to thrive
- Loss of muscle tone
- Bony abnormalities
- Breaking of blood vessels
- Limb edema (swelling)

Things that cause copper loss:[3, 4]
- Excess zinc
- Excess calcium
- Iron overload
- Fiber
- Excess molybdenum
- Antacid use
- Poor digestion
- Vegetarian diet
- Excess vitamin C
- Non-steroidal anti-inflammatory drugs e.g., aspirin, ibuprofen
- Penicillamine

Substances that increase copper:[5]
- Estrogens
- Environmental exposure in water pipes, cookware, birth control pills, and dental materials

Food Sources Of Copper:
Mg per 100 grams edible portion (100 grams = 3 ½ oz.)

13.7	Oysters	0.8	Buckwheat
2.3	Brazil nuts	0.8	Peanuts
2.1	Soy lecithin	0.7	Cod liver oil
1.4	Almonds	0.7	Lamb chops
1.3	Hazelnuts	0.5	Sunflower oil
1.3	Walnuts	0.4	Butter
1.3	Pecans	0.4	Rye grain
1.2	Split peas, dry	0.4	Pork loin
1.1	Beef liver	0.4	Barley

0.4	Gelatin	0.2	Chicken
0.3	Shrimp	0.2	Eggs
0.3	Olive oil	0.2	Corn oil
0.3	Clams	0.2	Ginger root
0.3	Carrots	0.2	Molasses
0.3	Coconut	0.2	Turnips
0.3	Garlic	0.1	Green peas
0.2	Millet	0.1	Papaya
0.2	Whole wheat	0.1	Apple

Reprinted with permission from *Clinical Nutrition: A Functional Approach* by Jeffrey Bland.[6]

Side effects: Abdominal pain, headaches, diarrhea, anemia, and liver, kidney, and brain damage can all occur if you take copper in excess.[7]

Dosage: 1.5 to 3.0 mg. *It is very important that copper and zinc stay in the right ratio to each other in your body.* The bioavailability of cupric oxide is almost zero and therefore it should not be used for treatment.[8]

8

Iodine

Iodine is added to many salts produced in the United States to prevent iodine deficiency. Sea salt is not as rich in iodine. Iodine is present in more than 100 enzyme systems in your body.

Functions of iodine in your body:[1, 2, 3]

- Needed for the development and functioning of the thyroid gland
- Maintains healthy breast tissue in women
- Fights bacteria
- Energy production
- Nerve function
- Hair and skin growth
- Protects against toxic effects from radioactive material
- Relieves pain and soreness associated with fibrocystic breast disease

Foods that interfere with iodine used by your thyroid:[4]

- Cabbage
- Rutabagas
- Cauliflower
- Soybeans

If you intake a large amount if these foods you may develop thyroid enlargement (goiter).

Food Sources Of Iodine:

Micrograms per 100 grams edible portion (100 grams = 3 ½ oz.)

90	Clams	11	Cheddar cheese
65	Shrimp	10	Pork
62	Haddock	10	Lettuce
50	Oysters	9	Spinach
50	Salmon	9	Green peppers
46	Halibut	9	Butter
37	Sardines, canned	7	Milk
19	Beef liver	6	Cream
16	Pineapple	6	Cottage cheese
16	Tuna, canned	6	Beef
14	Eggs	3	Lamb
11	Peanuts	3	Raisins
11	Whole wheat bread		

Reprinted with permission from *Clinical Nutrition: A Functional Approach* by Jeffrey Bland.[5]

Side effects: Acne-like skin lesions.[6]

Dosage: 150 micrograms

9

Iron

Functions of iron in your body:
- Is an essential component of blood (hemoglobin)
- Is needed for good cognition and behavior
- Involved in immune system health
- Key element in many enzymes
- Is needed for collagen synthesis

Symptoms of iron deficiency:[1, 2, 3, 4]
- Anemia (microcytic hypochromic)
- Fatigue
- Shortness of breath
- Rapid heart rate
- Pallor
- Headache
- Inflammation of the tongue
- Spoon nails
- Decreased cognitive function
- Craving for ice
- Short attention span
- Unhappiness
- Increased fearfulness
- Increased body tension
- Decreased immune system
- Impaired growth

- Increased blood sugar
- Hair loss
- Decreased memory
- Restless leg syndrome
- May increase the risk of jitteriness due to tricyclic antide-pressants

Causes of iron deficiency:[5, 6]

- Bleeding from any source
- Menstrual cycles
- Coffee
- Black tea
- Green tea
- Soy products
- Polyphenolic compounds
- Calcium
- Partially digested proteins

Things that increase iron absorption:[7]

- Vitamin C
- Cysteine
- Vitamin B6
- Folic acid
- Zinc

Foods Sources Of Iron:

Mg per 100 grams edible portion (100 grams = 3 ½ oz.)

100.0	Kelp	3.9	Dried prunes
17.3	Brewer's yeast	3.8	Cashews
16.1	Blackstrap molasses	3.7	Lean beef
14.9	Wheat bran	3.5	Raisins
11.2	Pumpkin and squash seeds	3.4	Jerusalem artichoke
9.4	Wheat germ	3.4	Brazil nuts
8.8	Beef liver	3.3	Beet greens
7.1	Sunflower seeds	3.2	Swiss chard
6.8	Millet	3.1	Dandelion greens
6.2	Parsley	3.1	English walnut
6.1	Clams	3.0	Dates
4.7	Almonds	2.9	Pork
		2.7	Cooked dry beans

2.4	Sesame seeds, hulled	0.8	Mushrooms
2.4	Pecans	0.7	Banana
2.3	Eggs	0.7	Beets
2.1	Lentils	0.7	Carrot
2.1	Peanuts	0.7	Eggplant
1.9	Lamb	0.7	Sweet potato
1.9	Tofu	0.6	Avocado
1.8	Green peas	0.6	Figs
1.6	Brown rice	0.6	Potato
1.6	Ripe olives	0.6	Corn
1.5	Chicken	0.5	Pineapple
1.3	Artichoke	0.5	Nectarine
1.3	Mung bean sprouts	0.5	Watermelon
1.2	Salmon	0.5	Winter squash
1.1	Broccoli	0.5	Brown rice, cooked
1.1	Currants	0.5	Tomato
1.1	Whole wheat bread	0.4	Orange
1.1	Cauliflower	0.4	Cherries
1.0	Cheddar cheese	0.4	Summer squash
1.0	Strawberries	0.3	Papaya
1.0	Asparagus	0.3	Celery
0.9	Blackberries	0.3	Cottage cheese
0.8	Red cabbage	0.3	Apple
0.8	Pumpkin		

Reprinted with permission from *Clinical Nutrition: A Functional Approach* by Jeffrey Bland.[8]

Side effects: *Excess levels of iron in your body can predispose you to heart disease.* Therefore, it is very important to take iron only if your doctor suggests that you need it. Also, too much iron is associated with an increase in free radical production and may increase your risk of cancer. Free radical production may also cause inflammation and make your arthritis symptoms worse. In addition, iron overload can cause diabetes and liver disease. Iron also decreases the absorption and utilization of vitamin E.[9]

Other symptoms of iron overload are hair loss and gut disturbances.

Dosage:
- Males: 10 mg
- Females: Pre-menopausal women: 15 mg
- Menopausal women need no additional iron unless instructed
  by their doctor.
- Pregnant women: 30 mg

Iron supplements can interfere with the absorption of the following medications:[10]
- Levothyroxine
- Ciprofloxacin
- Norfloxacin
- Captopril
- Penicillamine
- Blood thinners

10

Manganese

Functions of manganese in your body:[1]
- Essential for the utilization of vitamins B and C used in adrenal health
- Needed for the synthesis of cartilage, collagen, and other connective tissue
- Used for bone growth and maintenance
- Essential for a healthy nervous system and brain
- Used in blood formation
- Needed for a good immune system
- Required for the production of estrogen and progesterone
- Helps with carbohydrate metabolism
- Aids in protein digestion and synthesis
- Required for fatty acid synthesis
- Is a cofactor for enzymes involved in energy production
- Part of the antioxidant defense mechanism

Symptoms of deficiency:[2, 3]
- Impaired growth
- Impaired carbohydrate metabolism
- Decreased lipid metabolism
- Skeletal problems
- Loss of hair color
- Skin rash

- Decreased hair and nail growth
- Decreased HDL (good) cholesterol

What decreases manganese:[4]
- Phytates in bread
- Aluminum

Symptoms of excess manganese intake:[5]
- Disorientation
- Memory loss
- Anxiety
- Emotional lability
- Hallucinations
- Delusions
- Permanent brain damage

Food Sources Of Manganese:

Mg per 100 grams edible portion (100 grams = 3 ½ oz.)

3.5	Pecans	0.2	Cornmeal
2.8	Brazil nuts	0.2	Millet
2.5	Almonds	0.19	Gorgonzola cheese
1.8	Barley	0.16	Carrots
1.3	Rye	0.15	Broccoli
1.3	Buckwheat	0.14	Brown rice
1.3	Split peas, dry	0.14	Whole wheat bread
1.1	Whole wheat	0.13	Swiss cheese
0.8	Walnuts	0.13	Corn
0.8	Fresh spinach	0.11	Cabbage
0.7	Peanuts	0.10	Peach
0.6	Oats	0.09	Butter
0.5	Raisins	0.06	Tangerine
0.5	Turnip greens	0.06	Peas
0.5	Rhubarb	0.05	Eggs
0.4	Beet greens	0.04	Beets
0.3	Brussels sprouts	0.04	Coconut
0.3	Oatmeal	0.03	Apple

0.03 Orange
0.03 Pear
0.03 Lamb chops
0.03 Cantaloupe
0.03 Tomato
0.02 Whole milk
0.02 Chicken breasts

0.02 Green beans
0.02 Apricot
0.01 Beef liver
0.01 Scallops
0.01 Halibut
0.01 Cucumber

Cloves, ginger, thyme, bay leaves, and tea are also high in manganese.

Reprinted with permission from *Clinical Nutrition: A Functional Approach* by Jeffrey Bland.[6]

Side effects: *Use manganese with caution if you have gallbladder or liver disease.* Chronic inhalation of manganese by miners may be related to Parkinson's disease.[7]

Dosage: 2.5 to 5.0 mg

11

Molybdenum

Functions of molybdenum in your body:[1]
- Acts as a coenzyme in uric acid formation
- Acts as an electron transport agent in oxidation/reduction reactions
- Coenzyme in alcohol detoxification
- Used to detoxify sulfite

Symptoms of molybdenum deficiency:[2]
- Tachycardia (heart racing), headache, disorientation (symptoms of sulfite toxicity)

Food Sources Of Molybdenum:
Micrograms per 100 grams edible portion (100 grams = 3 ½ oz.)

155	Lentils	60	Oats
135	Beef liver	53	Eggs
130	Split peas	50	Rye bread
120	Cauliflower	45	Corn
110	Green peas	42	Barley
109	Brewer's yeast	40	Fish
100	Wheat germ	36	Whole wheat
100	Spinach	32	Whole wheat bread
77	Beef kidney	32	Chicken
75	Brown rice	31	Cottage cheese
70	Garlic	30	Beef

30	Potatoes	14	Apricots
25	Onions	10	Raisins
25	Coconut	10	Butter
25	Pork	7	Strawberries
24	Lamb	5	Carrots
21	Green beans	5	Cabbage
19	Crab	3	Whole milk
19	Molasses	1	Goat milk
16	Cantaloupe		

Reprinted with permission from *Clinical Nutrition: A Functional Approach* by Jeffrey Bland.[3]

Side effects: not toxic up to 9 mg a day. Above this dose molybdenum can cause symptoms similar to gout because of an increase in uric acid production.[4] Furthermore, excessive molybdenum intake may cause a copper deficiency.[5]

Dosage: 75-250 micrograms

Selenium

12

The selenium content of a food depends on what soil it is grown in. The selenium deficient states are: Connecticut, Illinois, Ohio, Oregon, Massachusetts, Rhode Island, New York, Pennsylvania, Indiana, and Delaware. Selenium levels are also low in the District of Columbia.[1] A study done at the Cleveland Clinic showed that people who live in states with low selenium content in their soil were three times more likely to die of heart disease than those who lived in states with adequate selenium content of their soil.[2]

Functions of selenium in your body:[3]
- Needed for immune system
- Works with vitamin E as an antioxidant
- Helps prevent cancer (has a role in DNA repair)
- Helps prevent heart disease
- Reduces heavy metal toxicity
- Involved in thyroid function

Manifestations of selenium deficiency:[4]
- Weakness
- Loss of pigment of skin and hair
- Skeletal muscle problems
- Thyroid enlargement
- Recurrent infections
- Low sperm counts

Low selenium levels occur in:[5]

- AIDS
- Inflammatory bowel disease
- Cancer
- Autoimmune disease
- Infertility (males)
- Thyroid disease

Food Sources Of Selenium:

Micrograms per 100 grams edible portion (100 grams = 3 ½ oz.)

146	Butter	25	Garlic
141	Smoked herring	24	Barley
123	Smelt	19	Orange juice
111	Wheat germ	19	Gelatin
103	Brazil nuts	19	Beer
89	Apple cider vinegar	18	Beef liver
77	Scallops	18	Lamb chop
66	Barley	18	Egg yolk
66	Whole wheat bread	12	Mushrooms
65	Lobster	12	Chicken
63	Bran	10	Swiss cheese
59	Shrimp	5	Cottage cheese
57	Red Swiss chard	5	Wine
56	Oats	4	Radishes
55	Clams	4	Grape juice
51	King crab	3	Pecans
49	Oysters	2	Hazelnuts
48	Milk	2	Almonds
43	Cod	2	Green beans
39	Brown rice	2	Kidney beans
34	Top round steak	2	Onion
30	Lamb	2	Carrots
27	Turnips	2	Cabbage
26	Molasses	1	Orange

Reprinted with permission form *Clinical Nutrition: A Functional Approach* by Jeffrey Bland.[6]

Symptoms of selenium toxicity:[7]

- Fatigue
- Irritability
- Dry hair
- Hair loss
- Nervous system problems
- Bad breath

Dosage: Do not take more than 200 micrograms a day unless directed by a physician.

13

Silicon

Function of silicon in your body:
- Responsible for skin, hair, and nail health
- Bone and cartilage development

Silicon is contained in apples, unrefined grains, legumes, rice bran, and root vegetables. Organic forms of silicon are found in stinging nettles and horsetail.

Side effects: None.

Dosage: 1-2 mg

14

Vanadium

Function of vanadium in your body:[1]
• Improves insulin sensitivity

Food Sources Of Vanadium:
Micrograms per 100 grams edible portion (100 grams = 3 ½ oz.)

100	Buckwheat	10	Cabbage
80	Parsley	10	Garlic
70	Soybeans	6	Tomatoes
64	Safflower oil	5	Radishes
42	Eggs	5	Onions
41	Sunflower seed oil	5	Whole wheat
35	Oats	4	Lobster
30	Olive oil	4	Beets
15	Sunflower seeds	3	Apples
15	Corn	2	Plums
14	Green beans	2	Lettuce
11	Peanut oil	2	Millet
10	Carrots		

Reprinted with permission from *Clinical Nutrition: A Functional Approach* by Jeffrey Bland.[2]

Symptoms of vanadium excess:[3]
- Elevated blood pressure
- Decreased coenzyme A
- Lower coenzyme Q-10
- Interference with cellular energy production

Side effects: *Bipolar disorder may be a toxic side effect.*[4] Consequently, do not take more than 50 mg a day without the supervision of a doctor.

Dosage: 10-50 mg

Zinc

15

Zinc is used in many enzymatic reactions in your body. One hundred enzymes need zinc as a cofactor.

Zinc has the following functions in your body:[1]
- Sexual maturation
- Fertility and reproduction
- Night vision
- Immune defenses
- Taste and appetite
- Metabolizes carbohydrates
- Helps balance blood sugar levels
- Decreases the requirement for insulin by the body
- Essential for DNA and RNA function needed for cell division and replication
- Is a structural part of your hormones
- Helps stabilize the cell membrane and structures in the cytoplasm of the cell
- Breaks down and metabolizes protein in the digestive system
- Helps assemble proteins inside the cell
- Needed for the formation of bone and skin
- Promotes thyroid activity
- Opposes toxic metals such as mercury
- Enhances the biochemical actions of vitamin D

- Is an antioxidant
- Is important for a healthy prostate
- Helps you absorb vitamin A
- Is needed for the proper maintenance of vitamin E
- Inhibits the enzyme that reduces levels of DHT (dihydrotestosterone)
- Promotes conversion of T4 to T3 (the more active form of thyroid)
- Anti-inflammatory

Symptoms of zinc deficiency:[2, 3, 4, 5]

- Hair loss
- Impaired wound healing
- Immune deficiencies
- Diarrhea
- Growth retardation
- Delayed sexual maturation
- Night blindness
- Behavioral disturbances (apathy, depression, irritability, confusion, hostile behavior)
- Low sperm count
- Anorexia
- Decreased sexual function
- Enlargement of the spleen and liver
- Dandruff
- Negative nitrogen balance
- Anemia
- Poor appetite
- Impaired nerve conduction and nerve damage
- Frontal headaches
- Crave sugary foods
- Decreased want for protein rich foods
- Sleep disturbances
- Acne
- Psoriasis
- Fatigue
- Decreased taste
- Brittle nails
- Eczema
- Decreased sense of smell
- White spots on nails
- Impotence
- Memory impairment
- Infertility
- Reduced salivation
- Stretch marks

Things that predispose you to zinc deficiency:[6, 7, 8]

- Alcoholism
- Pancreatitis
- Cirrhosis
- Inflammatory bowel disease
- Short bowel syndrome
- Chronic renal failure
- Anorexia nervosa
- Pancreatic insufficiency
- Cystic fibrosis
- Nephrotic syndrome
- Hemolytic anemia
- Celiac disease
- Surgery
- Infection
- Calcium
- Iron supplementation
- AIDS
- Smoking
- Aging (zinc absorption decreases with age)
- Rheumatoid arthritis
- Some diuretics

With each ejaculation a male loses 5 mg of zinc.[9] *The prostate needs 10 times more zinc than any other organ in the body.*

Food Sources Of Zinc:

Mg per 100 grams edible portion (100 grams = 3 ½ oz.)

148.7	Fresh oysters	3.0	Walnuts
6.8	Ginger root	2.9	Sardines
5.6	Ground round steak	2.6	Chicken
5.3	Lamb chops	2.5	Buckwheat
4.5	Pecans	2.4	Hazel nuts
4.2	Split peas, dry	1.9	Clams
4.2	Brazil nuts	1.7	Anchovies
3.9	Beef liver	1.7	Tuna
3.5	Nonfat dry milk	1.7	Haddock
3.5	Egg yolk	1.6	Green peas
3.2	Whole wheat	1.5	Shrimp
3.2	Rye	1.2	Turnips
3.2	Oats	0.9	Parsley
3.2	Peanuts	0.9	Potatoes
3.1	Lima beans	0.6	Garlic
3.1	Soy lecithin	0.5	Whole wheat bread
3.1	Almonds	0.4	Black beans

0.4	Raw milk	0.2	Lentils
0.4	Pork chop	0.2	Butter
0.4	Corn	0.2	Lettuce
0.3	Grape juice	0.1	Cucumber
0.3	Olive oil	0.1	Yams
0.3	Cauliflower	0.1	Tangerine
0.2	Spinach	0.1	String beans
0.2	Cabbage		

Black pepper, paprika, mustard chili powder, thyme, and cinnamon are also high in zinc.

Reprinted with permission from *Clinical Nutrition: A Functional Approach* by Jeffrey Bland.[10]

Things that interfere with the absorption of zinc:
- Tetracycline
- Cortisone
- Diuretics (water pills)
- Excess copper

Zinc decreases the absorption of:[11]
- Tetracycline
- Fluroquinolones

Side effects of too much zinc:[12]
- Decrease in immune system
- Premature heartbeats
- Dizziness
- Drowsiness
- Increased sweating
- Loss of muscular coordination
- Alcohol intolerance
- Hallucinations
- Anemia

Side effects: None below 100 mg.

Dosage: 25-50. The most well absorbed forms of zinc are zinc picolinate and zinc citrate.

Zinc is used to treat the following:[13]

- Acne
- Furuncles
- Eczema
- Colds
- Rheumatoid arthritis
- Gastric ulcers
- Macular degeneration
- Improve taste sensation
- Immune function
- Enlarged prostate
- Infertility
- Anorexia nervosa
- Diabetes mellitus
- Growth retardation
- Tinnitus

We used to think of vitamins strictly in terms of what is needed to prevent short-term deficiencies. Now we are starting to think about what is the optimal level of vitamins for lifelong health and to prevent age-associated diseases.

—Dr. Simin Meydani, Human Nutrition Research Center on Aging at Tufts University

Section 4

Fatty Acids

Your body requires fats to make your body work and prevent disease. The major shift in food consumption to a low fat diet deprives your body of essential fatty acids. Instead of eliminating fat from your diet you need to add "good" fats to your eating and nutrient supplementation program.

Fats occur in the following groups:

• Supersaturated/Omega-3-fatty acids

Alpha-linolenic acid occurs in flax, hemp seed, canola, soy bean, walnut, and dark green leaves

Stearidonic acid occurs in black currant seeds

Eicosapentaenoic acid (EPA) and docosahexaenoic acid (DHA) occurs in fish, nuts, and lamb

• Polyunsaturated/Omega-6-fatty acids

Linoleic acid occurs in safflower, sunflower, hemp, soybean, walnut, pumpkin, sesame, and flax oil

Gamma-linolenic acid (GLA) occurs in borage oil, black current seed, and evening primrose oil

Dihumogamma-linolenic acid (DGLA) occurs in mother's milk

Arachidonic acid occurs in meats and animal products

- Monounsaturated/Omega-9-fatty acids
    Oleic acid occurs in olive, almond, avocado, peanut, pecan, cashew, filbert, macadamia oils, butter, and animal fat
- Monounsaturated/Omega-7-fatty acid
    Palmitoleic acid occurs in coconut and palm oil
- Saturated fatty acids
    Stearic acid occurs in beef, mutton, pork, butter, and cocoa butter
    Palmitic acid occurs in coconut, palm, and palm kernel
    Butyric acid occurs in butter
    Arachidic acid occurs in peanuts

The omega-6-fatty acids produce inflammation and the omega-3-fatty acids decrease inflammation.

Functions of fatty acids in your body:[1, 2, 3, 4, 5]

- Provide structural support for the outer walls or membranes of the body's cells
- Help convert the nutrients from foods into usable forms of energy
- Involved in cell to cell communication
- Make it possible for nutrients to pass from the blood through the cell walls
- Helps with substance in the cells to pass into the blood
- Used to manufacture red blood cells
- Decreases inflammation
- Dilates or constricts blood vessels in the stomach, intestines, uterus, and bronchial tree
- Lowers triglycerides
- Makes blood less sticky
- Raises HDL (good) cholesterol
- Decreases arrhythmias (irregular heart rhythm)

- Decreased blood pressure
- May decrease homocysteine levels
- Enhances insulin action
- Helps protect against oxidation and ischemic heart disease
- Needed for normal development and function of your brain, eyes, inner ear, adrenal glands, and reproductive tract
- Needed to make prostaglandins I and II which decrease inflammation, increase immune function, and decrease menstrual cramps
- Reduces PMS symptoms
- Important for mitochondrial function (energy producing parts of your cells)

The following are clinical manifestations of essential fatty acid deficiency:[6, 7]

- Dry, scaly skin/dermatitis
- Dry hair, dandruff
- Brittle nails, graying with horizontal splitting
- Thirst, excess urination
- Decreased memory and mental abilities
- Psychological disturbances
- Impaired immune response
- Fatty infiltration of the liver
- Tingling or numbness of your arms or legs (neuropathy)
- Reduced vision
- Increased cholesterol
- Mood swings
- Depression
- Age-related memory declines
- Arthritis
- Asthma
- Slow wound healing
- Sterility in men
- Miscarriage
- Heart disease
- Hair Loss
- Cracking skin at finger tips
- Bumps on back of arms

There are two essential fats that your body cannot make by itself and you have to ingest them. They are linoleic acid (omega-6-fatty acid) and linolenic acid (omega-3-fatty acid). Neither of these groups of fatty acids can be made by your body and therefore they must be eaten or taken as a supplement.

Your body requires omega-6-fatty acids to maintain your health. However if you intake too many of them you cause inflammation by producing prostaglandins that go down an inflammatory pathway instead of an anti-inflammatory pathway. The standard American diet is very low in omega-3-fatty acids and very high in omega-6-fatty acids. It is best to intake three to six parts of omega-6 fatty acids to one part omega-3-fatty acids instead of what most Americans eat which is between 10:1 to 25:1.[8]

Your body requires zinc, magnesium, niacin, vitamin C, vitamin A, biotin, B vitamins, and other nutrients to convert fatty acids.[9]

What causes a deficiency of fatty acids in your body:[10]
- Decrease intake of the right kind of fatty acids
- Stress
- Inability to absorb fatty acids
- Alcoholism
- Type I diabetes
- Decrease intake of nutrients needed as cofactors
- Carnitine deficiency
- Increase in trans fatty acid intake (interferes with fatty acid synthesis)
- Increase in sugar intake (interferes with the enzymes of fatty acid synthesis)

Diseases treated by fatty acids:[11, 12, 13, 14, 15, 16, 17, 18, 19, 20, 21, 22, 23, 24, 25, 26, 27, 28, 29, 30, 31, 32, 33, 34, 35, 36, 37, 38, 39, 40, 41, 42, 43]

- Heart disease (prevent and treat)
- High triglycerides
- High blood pressure
- Depression
- Arthritis (rheumatoid and osteo)
- Psoriasis
- Autoimmune disorders
- Crohn's disease
- Helps to prevent cancer of the breast, colon, lung, skin, and prostate
- Diabetes (prevent and treat)
- Asthma

- Irritable bowel
- Irregular heart rhythms
- Increases memory and decreases cognitive decline
- Eczema
- Benign familial tremor
- Neuropathy
- Schizophrenia
- Bipolar illness
- Ulcerative colitis
- High cholesterol
- Enlarged prostate
- Constipation
- Multiple Sclerosis
- Parkinson's disease
- ADD/ADHD
- Menopause (hot flashes)
- Menstrual cramps
- Migraine headaches
- Weight loss
- Alzheimer's disease
- Prevent memory decline
- Chronic fatigue syndrome
- PMS
- Eye disease (retinal)
- Stroke (prevention, recovery)
- Anorexia nervosa
- Aggression
- Autism
- Brain tumor (glioma)
- Cerebral palsy
- Developmental delay
- Down's syndrome
- Drug abuse
- Head injury
- Numbness and tingling
- Phobias
- Postpartum depression

Fatty acid intake can change the amount of medication that you may need. You may require less Prozac or insulin, for example.[44] *If you are taking blood thinners then consult your doctor concerning the amount of fatty acids you should intake.*

Fatty acids can become rancid and therefore should be refrigerated. *Take vitamin E when using omega-3-fatty acids to prevent oxidation.* Some people experience burping up of fatty acids. This can be avoided by putting them in the freezer prior to use. This does not destroy their effectiveness. Have your doctor measure your essential and metabolic fatty acids. This test is available through Great Smokies Laboratory (see Appendix).

Trans fatty acids do not occur naturally in nature. They were developed by the food industry to help food stay fresh longer. They have been shown to increase LDL (bad cholesterol), decrease HDL (good cholesterol), increase triglycerides, increase lipoprotein (a), and make platelets sticker which increases blood clots. Furthermore, trans fatty acids cause your cell membranes to leak, disrupting cellular metabolism and allowing toxins to enter your cells.[45] All processed oils contain trans fatty acids. Consequently do not use processed oils. The more solid the oil, the more trans fatty acids included in it. Liquid vegetable oils contain up to 6 percent trans fats and margarines and shortening up to 58 percent trans fatty acids.[46] In Europe there are mandates against trans fatty acids. *Anything that says hydrogenated or partially hydrogenated contains trans fatty acids. Trans fatty acids will increase your risk of heart disease. Furthermore, trans fatty acids interfere with your body's ability to make its own DHA.*[47]

Trans fatty acids occur in:[48]

- Boxed foods
- Breads
- Candies
- Chocolate
- Frozen diners
- Processed meats
- French fries
- Potato chips
- Corn chips/tortilla chips
- Donuts
- Pastries
- Margarine
- Mayonnaise

*Nutrients are found together
in nature and work in the
body as a team.*
—Roger Williams, Ph.D.

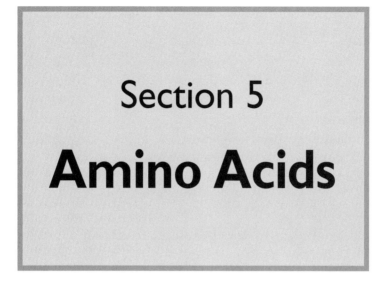

Section 5

Amino Acids

Proteins are made up of amino acids. They function as the building blocks of muscle and comprise all of the body's enzymes and many of its peptides. Proteins are also one of the sources of energy in your body and promote repair of damaged tissue.

When you eat protein your body breaks it down into amino acids and peptides. It is the amino acids that are the nutritional part of the protein that provides function. There are 40,000 different proteins found in your body and they are all made from 20 amino acids. Some are essential amino acids. These are the ones that your system cannot manufacture on their own. Other amino acids are nonessential. These can be made in sufficient quantities by your own body. A third kind of amino acids is called conditionally essential amino acids. Under normal conditions in your body you are able to make them. However, when you have a fever, illness, are dieting, or are getting chemotherapy, you cannot make some of these amino acids. Furthermore, your body may be using up all of its essential amino acids in detoxifying or repairing and then you will still need to ingest them even though your body is able to make them. Many phase II detoxi-fication reactions use amino acids (see chapter on detoxification).

Essential	Conditionally Essential	Nonessential
Histidine	Arginine	Alanine
Isoleucine	Cysteine	Arginine
Leucine	Cystine	Aspartic acid
Lysine	Glutamine	Asparagine
Methionine	Taurine	Glutamic acid
Phenylalanine	Tyrosine	Glycine
Threonine		Proline
Tryptophan		Serine
Valine		

Your body also makes other amino acids that are not usually included in the above grouping such as GABA (gamma aminobutyric acid, acetyl-L-carnitine, glutathione, and homocysteine) which will be discussed elsewhere in this book. For further reading, a great book on this subject is *Heal with Amino Acids and Nutrients* by Dr. Billie Sahley.[1]

This section of the text will focus on some of the essential, conditionally essential, and nonessential amino acids. It is not designed to be a comprehensive text of this subject. *If you have kidney or liver disease you should consult a physician before taking any amino acid supplement.*

Symptoms of amino acid deficiencies:[2]
- Chronic fatigue
- Food/chemical allergies
- Recurrent ear infections
- Frequent colds
- Mental/emotional problems
- Hyperactivity
- Depression
- Anxiety
- Frequent headaches

- Insomnia
- Mood swings
- ADD/ADHD
- Immune dysfunction
- Neurological disorders
- Blood sugar disorders
- Arthritis
- PMS
- Alcoholism
- Obsessive compulsive disorder (OCD)
- Aggressive behavior
- Carbohydrate and sugar cravings
- Panic attacks
- Fibromyalgia

The dosages of amino acids are best delineated by having your physician order an amino acid analysis test (see Appendix under Great Smokies Diagnostic Laboratory for availability). Then have your doctor contact a compounding pharmacist near you to have your amino acid formulation made up as a prescription especially if your lab work reveals that you are deficient in several amino acids (see Appendix under PCCA for a pharmacy near you). Likewise, any of the pharmaceutical grade companies that offer amino acids are also a good place for you and your physician to begin if you are deficient in one or two amino acids (see Appendix). *If you are taking amino acids you need to also be taking vitamin B6 to help your body metabolize them.*

Alanine

Alanine requires vitamin B6 for metabolism.

Functions of alanine in your body:[1]
- Is an inhibitory neurotransmitter in the brain
- Is needed to metabolize tryptophan

Food sources of alanine are wheat germ, turkey, duck, cottage cheese, and sausage.[2]

Dosage: 200-600 mg

Arginine

2

Arginine promotes the following functions in your body:[1, 2, 3, 4, 5]

- Increases immune function by increasing natural killer cell activity
- Inhibits plaque accumulation in your arteries
- Increases circulation
- Increases growth hormone production
- Builds muscle
- Enhances fat metabolism
- Increases sperm count
- Enhances immune function
- Needed for protein production
- Vital for secretion of glucagons and insulin
- Important for gut health
- Reduces pain from claudication (poor circulation)
- Helps wounds heal
- Decreases platelet stickiness

Symptoms associated with arginine deficiency:[6]

- Skin rash
- Hair loss and breakage
- Poor wound healing
- Constipation
- Fatty liver
- Hepatic cirrhosis
- Coma
- Hypoglycemia

Natural sources of arginine are in beans, brewer's yeast, chocolate, dairy products, eggs, fish, legumes, meat, nuts, oatmeal, popcorn, raisins, seafood, seeds, sesame seeds, soy, sunflower seeds, whey, green peas, asparagus, broccoli, Swiss chard, corn, potatoes, onion, spinach, avocados, and whole grains.[7, 8]

Side effects: Supplementation may cause an increase in herpes simplex infections (cold sores).

Dosage: 1,000-3,000 mg

3

Aspargine

***Functions of aspargine:*[1]**
- Helps protect the liver
- Promotes mineral uptake in the intestinal tract
- Helps ammonia detoxify
- Metabolizes carbohydrates via the Krebs cycle
- Forms part of DNA

Food sources of aspargine include pork, turkey, sausage, chicken, wheat germ, cottage and ricotta cheeses.[2]

Dosage: according to lab results.

4

Cysteine

Cysteine is a nonessential amino acid that is made in your liver. N-acetyl cysteine (NAC) is a modified form of cysteine and aids your body in making the strong antioxidant glutathione.

Cysteine has the following functions in your body:[1]

- Helps protect against heart disease
- Aids in cancer protection (stimulates natural killer cells)
- Boosts your immune system
- Promotes metabolism of fats and production of muscle
- Aids in healing after surgery
- Is an antioxidant
- Promotes hair growth
- Prevents hair loss
- Involved in communication between cells
- Breaks down homocysteine
- Reduces inflammation
- Helps destroy acetaldehyde and free radicals produced by smoking and drinking

You can get cysteine from beans, brewer's yeast, broccoli, Brussels sprouts, dairy products, eggs, fish, garlic, legumes, meat, nuts, onions, red peppers, seafood, seeds, soy, whey, and whole grains.[2]

Side effects: Cysteine supplements must be taken with vitamin C to prevent cysteine from being converted and increasing kidney stone production[3] You also cannot use cysteine if you have an active peptic ulcer.[4] Furthermore, if you are diabetic you should not use cysteine since it may cause glucose levels to change.[5]

Side effects of cysteine:[6]

- Nausea
- Vomiting
- Abdominal pain
- Indigestion
- Dyspepsia
- Dry mouth
- Headache
- Dizziness
- Flushes
- Sweating
- Blurred vision
- Abnormal taste
- Skin rash
- Anorexia
- Diarrhea
- Shortness of breath
- Asthma
- Constipation

5

Glutamine

Functions of glutamine in your body: [1, 2, 3, 4, 5, 6, 7, 8]

- Needed for the metabolism and maintenance of muscle
- Is a fuel source for your immune system
- Needed for DNA synthesis
- Promotes wound healing and tissue repair
- Neutralizes toxins
- Needed for a healthy gut
- Supports glutathione
- Promotes growth
- Stops food cravings
- Promotes weight loss
- Promotes a healthy acid-alkaline balance in your body
- Is an inhibitory neurotransmitter
- Increases energy
- Improves mental alertness
- Helps the brain dispose of ammonia
- Fights cold and flu
- Balances blood sugar
- Increases growth hormone
- Protects the body from stress
- Is a precursor for GABA

Food sources of glutamine are in beans, brewer's yeast, brown rice, dairy products, eggs, fish, legumes, meat, nuts, seafood, seeds, soy, whey, and whole grains.[9]

Dosage: 500-3,000 mg

Side effects: *If you have a sensitivity to MSG (monosodium glutamate) you should use glutamine with caution because your body metabolizes glutamine into glutamate. If you are taking medications for seizures only take glutamine under the direction of your doctor.*[10]

6

Glycine

Functions of glycine in your body:[1, 2]
- Is important in the manufacture of glucose from glycogen in your liver
- Used in the synthesis of hemoglobin, glutathione, DNA, and RNA
- Needed to maintain the nervous system
- Enhances the neurotransmitters (messengers) in your brain/ inhibitory neurotransmitter
- Needed for prostate gland function
- Helps form collagen
- Involved in the metabolism of bile salts
- Used for the formation of glutathione
- Helps detoxify heavy metals from your body
- Calms aggression
- Decreases sugar cravings
- Used in metabolism of proteins

Glycine is naturally found in meats and wheat germ.[3]

Side effects: *If you are taking clozapine or a related medication you should not take glycine.*[4]

Dosage: 500-3,000 mg

7

Histidine

Functions of histidine in your body:[1, 2]
- Needed for the maintenance of the myelin sheaths in your nervous system
- Dilates vessels
- Is a mild anti-inflammatory
- Produces histamine
- Helps to chelate minerals

Food sources of histidine are meats, chicken, turkey, fish, beans (especially soy), cheese, milk, eggs, grains, nuts, seeds, cereals, potatoes.[3]

Dosage: according to lab results.

8

Lysine

Lysine has the following functions in your body:[1, 2]

- Helps support immune defense
- Helps fight herpes outbreaks (cold sores)
- Helps maintain bone health by enhancing calcium absorption
- Helps protect the lens of the eye
- Regulates the pineal gland, mammary glands, and ovaries
- Required for growth and tissue repair
- Needed from production of hormones
- Aids in the production of antibodies
- Needed for making enzymes
- Increases growth hormone
- Maintains nitrogen balance
- Used in collagen production

Symptoms of lysine deficiency:[3, 4]

- Fatigue
- Inability to concentrate
- Irritability
- Bloodshot eyes
- Retarded growth
- Anemia
- Hair loss
- Apathy
- Depression
- Edema (swelling)
- Fever blisters
- Infertility
- Loss of energy
- Muscle loss
- Stomach ulcers
- Weakness

Sources of lysine include beans, brewer's yeast, cheese, dairy products, eggs, fish, legumes, lima beans, meat, green peas, asparagus, broccoli, corn, mushrooms, spinach, avocado, chocolate, nuts, potatoes, seafood, seeds, soy, whey, whole grains, and yeast.[5, 6]

Side effects: Lysine should not be taken for more than 6 months since it can cause an imbalance of arginine. *If you are allergic to eggs, milk, or wheat, or have diabetes you should not take lysine.*[7]

Dosage: 500-1,600 mg. If outbreaks of herpes occur, increase the amount to 3,000 mg a day until the outbreak has resolved.

9

Methionine

Functions of methionine in your body:[1, 2]

- Needed for the absorption, transportation, and availability of zinc and selenium
- Facilitates the breakdown of fats
- Prevents fat accumulation in your liver and arteries
- Normalizes homocysteine
- Needed for the formation of nucleic acids, epinephrine, choline, lecithin, carnitine, melatonin, collagen, serine, and creatine.
- Detoxifies the body of heavy metals

Symptoms of methionine deficiency:[3]

- Apathy
- Loss of pigmentation in hair
- Edema (swelling)
- Lethargy
- Liver damage
- Muscle loss
- Fat loss
- Skin lesions
- Weakness
- Slow growth in children

Food sources of methionine include sunflower seeds, pork, sausage, eggs, duck, wild game, lentils, pumpkin, avocado, cottage cheese, cheese, seafood, whey, and wheat germ.[4]

Side effects: If you are taking methionine always add B6 and folic acid to prevent a buildup of homocysteine.

Dosage: 1,000-2,000 mg

Phenylalanine 10

Phenylalanine converts to tyrosine in the liver. Tyrosine is then converted into the neurotransmitters L-dopa, norepinephrine, and epinephrine.

Functions of phenylalanine:[1, 2]

- Aids in thyroid hormone formation
- Improves mood, alertness, and ambition
- Regulates the release of cholecystokin (CCK), the hormone that signals the brain to feel satisfied after eating

Symptoms of phenylalanine deficiency:[3]

- Low levels of proteins
- Apathy
- Loss of pigmentation in hair
- Edema (swelling)
- Lethargy
- Liver damage
- Muscle loss
- Fat loss
- Skin lesions
- Weakness

Food sources of phenylalanine are almonds, avocado, bananas, beans, brewer's yeast, cheese, corn, dairy products, eggs, fish, lentils, sweet potatoes, potatoes, spinach, corn, green peas, Swiss chard, avocado, legumes, lima beans, nuts, meat, pickled herring, pumpkin seeds, sesame seeds, soy, whey, chocolate, and whole grains.[4, 5]

Side effects: *Phenylalanine should not be taken if you have the disease phenylketonuria (PKU) or if you are taking MAO inhibitors or tricyclic antidepressants. You should also not use tyrosine.*

Dosage: 500-3,000 mg

11

Proline

Proline can be manufactured in your body from ornithine or glutamic acid. It is needed for the formation of collagen but requires that vitamin C be present.

Food sources of proline include cottage and ricotta cheeses, eggs, pork, luncheon meats, wheat germ, turkey, and duck.[1]

Dosage: according to lab results.

Serine

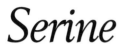

Serine is made from glycine with folic acid and vitamin B6.

Functions of serine in your body:[1, 2]
- Needed for DNA synthesis
- Used in the formation of neurotransmitters
- Stabilizes cell membranes
- Needed for the metabolism of fats and fatty acids
- Aids in muscle growth
- Helps maintain a healthy immune system
- Plays a part in the production of immunoglobulins and antibodies
- Has a role in the manufacture of nerve cell sheath

Dosage: according to lab results.

13

Taurine

Taurine requires zinc to help it function properly. In an adult, taurine is a conditionally essential amino acid and is made from methionine and cysteine. In children, it is an essential amino acid and must be taken in. It is required for normal brain development. Stress depletes your body of taurine.

Functions of taurine in your body:[1, 2, 3, 4, 5, 6, 7, 8]

- Lowers blood pressure
- Boosts antioxidant defense
- Supports immune system
- Strengthens the heart muscle
- Stabilizes heart rhythm
- Prevents blood clots
- Aids in glucose metabolism by increasing the activity of the insulin receptor
- Improves sensitivity to insulin
- Is a natural diuretic
- Improves lung health
- Protects cell membranes from damage
- Detoxifies toxic substances
- Needed for kidney function
- Needed for the formation of bile acids
- Is an inhibitory neurotransmitter
- Helps modulate calcium movement

- Aids wound healing
- Stabilizes membranes
- Improves fat metabolism in the liver

Symptoms of taurine deficiency:[9]

- Anxiety
- Seizures
- Hyperactivity
- Impaired brain function

Taurine is used in the treatment of:[10, 11, 12, 13, 14, 15, 16, 17, 18, 19]

- Macular degeneration
- Diabetes
- Epilepsy
- Congestive heart failure
- High blood pressure
- Decreases platelet stickiness
- Iron deficiency anemia
- Psoriasis
- Wound healing
- During chemotherapy and radiation

Foods that contain taurine are brewer's yeast, dairy products, eggs, fish, meat, and seafood.

Side effects: *Taurine should not be taken with aspirin or any salicylates.*

Dosage: 1-4 grams. Your requirement for taurine increases when you are stressed or ill.

If your homocysteine level is high you may have a block in the pathway that makes taurine.

14

Threonine

Functions of threonine in your body:[1]
- Needed for the formation of tooth enamel, collagen, and elastin
- Helps to metabolize fat
- Prevents the buildup of fat in the liver
- Stabilizes blood sugar
- Needed for proper digestion

Food sources include beans, brewer's yeast, dairy products, eggs, fish, legumes, meat, nuts, seafood, seeds, soy, whey, corn, green peas, potatoes, spinach, and whole grains.[2, 3]

Dosage: according to lab results.

Tryptophan 15

Typtophan works best if taken with B6 and carbohydrates. Your body requires B6 to make tryptophan. It has just recently become available again without a prescription.

Functions of tryptophan:[1, 2]
- Breaks down into serotonin, your calming neurotransmitter
- Acts as a mood stabilizer
- Helps with insomnia
- Boosts the release of growth hormone
- Suppresses your appetite
- Needed for the production of vitamin B3
- Is an inhibitory neurotransmitter

Foods that contain tryptophan are turkey, chicken, pork, meats, fish, beans, dairy products, eggs, grains, cereals, nuts, and seeds.[3]

Side effects: *If you are taking SSRIs or MAO inhibitors for depression, you should not take tryptophan.*

Dosage: 5-50 mg

16
5-HTP (5-hydroxytryptophan)

Functions of 5-HTP:
- Manufactures the neurotransmitter serotonin

5-HTP is used to treat the following:[1, 2, 3, 4, 5]
- Depression
- Fibromyalgia
- Chronic headaches
- Insomnia
- Pain management
- Anxiety
- Hyperactivity
- Stress
- PMS
- Obsessive/compulsive disorder
- Addiction
- Carbohydrate cravings

Side effects: If you are taking SSRIs or other antidepressant you should not take 5-HTP. If you are taking medication for Parkinson's disease you should not take 5-HTP.

Dosage: 50-300 mg. Magnesium prolongs the benefits of 5-HTP.

Tyrosine

17

Tyrosine becomes the neurotransmitters L-dopa, dopamine, norepinephrine, and epinephrine in your body.

Functions of tyrosine in your body:
- Helps form melanin, your skin pigment
- Aids in making one of the thyroid hormones, thyroxin
- Helps you deal with stress
- Is an inhibitor neurotransmitter

Symptoms of tyrosine deficiency include:[1]
- Apathy
- Blood sugar imbalances
- Depression
- Edema (swelling)
- Fat loss
- Fatigue
- Lethargy
- Liver damage
- Loss of pigmentation in hair
- Low serum levels of essential proteins
- Mood disorders
- Muscle loss
- Skin lesions
- Slowed growth in children
- Stress
- Weakness

Foods that contain tyrosine include almonds, avocados, bananas, beans, brewer's yeast, cheese, cottage cheese, dairy products, eggs, fish, legumes, lima beans, meat, milk, nuts, pickled herring, pumpkin seeds, corn, potatoes, spinach, nuts, seafood, seeds, soy, whey, and whole grains.[2, 3]

Dosage: 500-2,000 mg

Side effects: hypertension (high blood pressure), hypotension (low blood pressure), and migraine headaches. *Do not use if you are taking a MAO inhibitor medication.*[4]

*Nutrition has been
the 'missing link'
in modern medicine.*
—Jack Challem, Author
of *Syndrome X*

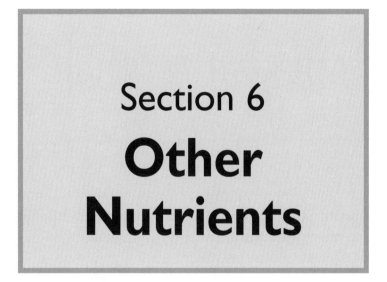

Section 6
Other Nutrients

This section of the book will look at individual nutrients not previously discussed. *Please consult your physician before taking any of the supplements described in this book if you have kidney or liver disease, are pregnant, or nursing.*

Ashwaganda Root (Withania somniferum)

1

Ashwaganda is an herb that has the following properties:[1, 2]
- Activates your immune system
- Helps preserve adrenal size
- Helps you deal with stress
- Increases muscle mass
- Enhances endurance and strength
- Lowers cholesterol
- Anti-inflammatory
- Protects your liver
- Antibacterial
- Antioxidant
- Increases libido and sexual performance

Dosage: 500-2,000 mg

2

Bilberry
(Vaccinium myrtillus)

Bilberry is a member of the same genus as the blueberry. The active component is part of the concentrated fruit pigments called "anthocyanins." Bilberry also contains tannins and vitamins A and C.

Bilberry has the following properties:[1]
- Improves circulation
- Slows the progression of cataracts
- Reduces the effects of diabetic retinopathy
- Antibacterial
- Antiviral
- Helps your eyes adapt to the dark

Dosage: 60-280 mg

3

CLA

CLA is a naturally occurring fatty acid.

Functions of CLA:[1, 2, 3, 4, 5, 6, 7, 8]

- Helps fight cancer
- Is an antioxidant
- Lowers cholesterol
- Builds immune system
- Improves insulin sensitivity
- Aids in weight loss

Dosage:

- Preventive: 100-500 mg
- Weight loss: 3,000-4,000 mg

4

L-Carnitine

L-carnitine is an amino acid. It is made from lysine and methionine in your liver, kidneys, and brain. Therefore if you are deficient in carnitine you also lack enough lysine and methionine. You also must have enough niacin, vitamin B6, iron, and vitamin C to make carnitine.

Functions of carnitine in your body:[1, 2, 3, 4, 5, 6]
- Needed for the transport of long-chain fatty acids into the cells
- Helps convert stored body fat into energy
- Energizes the heart
- Reduces triglycerides
- Lowers cholesterol
- Raises HDL (good cholesterol)
- May slow the progression of Alzheimer's disease
- Prevents DNA degeneration
- Promotes DNA repair from mutations that occur from free radical production
- Reduces the build up of acids and metabolic waste
- Increases oxygen availability and respiratory efficiency
- Can be converted to acetyl choline in your body
- Improves mental focus and energy
- Enhances short and long term memory

Things that can cause a deficiency of carnitine:[7]

- Deficiency of vitamin C, B6, or B12
- Deficiency of folic acid
- Iron deficiency
- Deficiency of SAMe
- Lysine deficiency
- Valproic acid
- Pivampicillin
- Ipecac syrup
- Sulfadiazine
- Pyrimethamine
- Vegetarian diet

Side effects: rare. They include skin rash, increased appetite, nausea, vomiting, dizziness, headache, agitation, and body odor (which is prevented by taking riboflavin). *If you have liver or kidney disease you should contact your physician before starting on carnitine.*

Carnitine is effective in the treatment of:[8, 9, 10, 11, 12, 13, 14, 15]

- Brain injuries and stroke
- Memory enhancement
- Alzheimer's disease
- Senility
- Depression
- Nerve injury
- Immune enhancement
- Angina
- Post heart attack
- Congestive heart failure
- Increased cholesterol
- Increased triglycerides
- Infertility
- Mitral valve prolapse
- ADD
- Weight loss
- Parkinson's disease

These nutrients help carnitine work more effectively:

- Phosphatidylserine
- B vitamins
- Alpha lipoic acid
- Phosphatidyl choline
- EPA/DHA

Dosage: 500-4,000 mg. Acetyl-L-carnitine is the form of carnitine that is effective in maintaining memory and stroke recovery.

5

Carnosine

Carnosine is an amino acid that is a combination of beta-alanine and histidine. *Do not confuse this nutrient with carnitine!* Carnosine protects your body from one of the main events responsible for aging called glycation. Proteins that are glycated produce more free radicals than nonglycated proteins.

Functions of carnosine in your body:[1, 2, 3, 4, 5]
- Is an antioxidant
- Binds metal ions that cause tissue damage
- Blocks the aging effects of glycation
- Helps maintain memory

Dosage: 1,000-2,000 mg

Side effects: *If you have kidney or liver disease, contact your doctor before taking carnosine.*

Carnosine is used in the treatment of:[6, 7, 8, 9, 10, 11, 12, 13]
- Alzheimer's disease
- Aging
- Atherosclerosis
- Brain injury
- Cataracts
- Diabetes mellitus
- Hypertension
- Stroke
- Wound healing

Coenzyme Q-10

6

Coenzyme Q-10 is a fat-soluble nutrient. It is made in almost every tissue in you body, however the amount that you make declines with age.

Functions of coenzyme Q-10:[1]

- Is an antioxidant
- Is a coenzyme in the energy-producing metabolic pathways of *all* of your cells
- Enhances the regeneration of vitamin E
- Reduces platelet stickiness
- Lowers blood pressure

What causes a deficiency of Q-10?[2, 3, 4, 5]

- Insufficient dietary intake
  - Taurine deficiency
- Impaired synthesis
  - Folic acid deficiency
  - Deficiency of vitamins B1, B12, B6, B5
- Drug interactions

Glucophage	Clonidine
Glyburide	Fluphenizine
Beta blockers	Hydroclorothiazide
Adriamycin	Simvistatin
Phenothiazines	Desipramine
Gemfibrozil	Fluvastatin

Haloperidol   Doxepin
Imipramine   Hydralizine
Provastatin   Lovastatin
Tolazemide   Protryptyline
Chlorpromazine   Trimipramine

- Exercise
- Hyperthyroidism
- Malabsorption
    Sprue
    Coeliac disease
    Steatorrhea (fatty stools)

Coenzyme Q-10 is effective in the treatment and prevention of:[6, 7, 8, 9, 10, 11, 12, 13, 14, 15]

- Coronary heart disease (heart disease)
- Arrhythmia (abnormal heart rhythm)
- High blood pressure
- Side effects of adriamycin treatment
- Parkinson's disease
- Alzheimer's disease
- Diabetes
- COPD (chronic obstructive pulmonary disease)
- Pulmonary fibrosis
- Asthma
- Periodontal disease
- Weight loss
- Sun damaged skin
- Congestive heart failure
- Dilated cardiomyopathy
- Migraine headaches
- Chronic fatigue/fibromyalgia
- Mitral valve prolapse

Side effects of Q-10:[16]

- Insomnia (in doses greater than 100 mg)
- Palpitations
- Diarrhea
- Appetite loss
- Mild nausea
- Increase in liver enzymes (in doses greater than 300 mg)
- Abdominal discomfort
- Photophobia
- Irritability
- Heartburn

If you take coenzyme Q-10 after meals the side effects are lessened.

Dosage: 30-360 mg depending on diagnosis. Do not use more than 100 mg without consulting a health care provider.

Side effects: *Coenzyme Q-10 should not be used without the close supervision of your doctor if you are taking a blood thinner.*

Foods that contain coenzyme Q-10 include beef heart, pork, sardines, anchovies, mackerel, salmon, broccoli, spinach, and nuts.

Statin drugs deplete your body of coenzyme Q-10 which some studies have shown may make a woman more vulnerable to breast cancer. These medications include Lipitor, Mevacor, Zocor, Pravachol, and others that are in a class of drugs called HMG-CoA-reductase inhibitors.[17] *Therefore, if you are a woman and taking a statin drug, you should take at least 100 mg a day of coenzyme Q-10.*

I believe that no single factor plays a more significant role in the origin of disease—or in its cure or prevention—than obtaining sufficient dietary fiber.

—Ted Broer, Ph.D., Author
of *Maximum Energy*

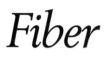

Fiber

Fiber is a food substance found in plants that contains no nutrients or calories. They are not digested or absorbed by your body.

Benefits of fiber:[1, 2]

- Prevents constipation
- Lowers blood sugar
- Lowers cholesterol
- Lowers blood pressure
- Lowers triglycerides
- Increases HDL

Fiber occurs in both a soluble and insoluble form.

Soluble fiber binds to fats in foods and prevents their absorption which helps lower your cholesterol.

Sources of soluble fiber:[3]

- Apples
- Apricots
- Bananas
- Chick peas
- Oat bran
- Broccoli
- Psyllium
- Barley
- Cabbage
- Flax seed
- Nuts
- Okra
- Oranges
- Grapefruit
- Pears
- Pinto, navy, lima, and kidney beans
- Prunes
- Split peas
- Sweet potatoes

Insoluble fiber speeds up movement of food through your body.

Sources of insoluble fiber:[4]

- Grains
- Beans
- Celery
- Corn
- Lentils
- High-fiber cereal
- Potato (with skin)
- Wheat bran
- Prunes
- Bananas
- Broccoli
- Brown rice
- Brussels sprouts
- Cauliflower
- Spinach
- Wheat bran (unprocessed)
- Whole wheat bread
- Pasta
- Crackers

8

GABA

GABA is an amino acid. It is found in large amounts in the area of your brain known as the hypothalamus. When you use GABA it is important that you also take vitamin B6 to act as a cofactor. Otherwise, your body cannot metabolize GABA properly.

Functions of GABA:[1, 2]

- Is an inhibitory neurotransmitter
- Produces a calming affect on the brain
- Aids your body in secreting growth hormone
- Muscle relaxant
- Lowers blood pressure
- Helps control hypoglycemia
- Prevents anxiety
- Promotes sleep

Symptoms of GABA deficiency:[3]

- Anxiety
- Sensation that your brain is racing out of control

Foods that contain GABA are beans, brewer's yeast, dairy products, eggs, fish, legumes, meat, nuts, seafood, seeds, soy, whey, and whole grains.[4]

Side effects: Some people experience a tingling sensation in the face and a slight shortness of breath after taking GABA which will last for only a few minutes. If GABA makes you drowsy, then take in the evening. *If you have kidney or liver disease, contact your physician before you take GABA.*

Dosage:

- If you weigh less than 125 pounds, 375 mg three times a day.
- If you weigh more than 125 pounds, 750 mg three times a day.

Garlic (Allium sativum) 9

The main active ingredient in garlic is allicin. Garlic contains amino acids, vitamins, trace minerals, flavonoids, enzymes, and 200 additional compounds.

Benefits of garlic:[1, 2, 3, 4, 5, 6, 7, 8, 9, 10, 11]

- Lowers triglycerides
- Decreases LDL (bad) cholesterol
- Raises HDL (good) cholesterol
- Increases your immune system (acts as antibiotic, antiviral, antifungal agent)
- Balances blood sugar
- Reduces the risk of developing esophageal, stomach, and colon cancer
- May lower risk of prostate cancer
- Natural blood thinner
- Lowers blood pressure
- Increases nitric oxide
- Boosts natural killer cell activity (helps prevent cancer)

Dosage: Garlic products are described in terms of fresh or whole garlic equivalent. An average dose is 1,500-1,800 mg of fresh garlic equivalent which equals one-half a clove of fresh garlic.

Side effects: *Garlic is a blood thinner. Check with your physician if you are taking a blood thinner before taking large amounts of garlic. If you are pregnant do not take large doses of garlic since it may cause uterine contractions.*

Ginkgo

10

Ginkgo biloba is an herbal extract from the leaves of the ginkgo tree.

Benefits of ginkgo:[1]

- Is an antioxidant and prevents membrane damage
- Increases oxygen to the brain by increasing blood supply (dilates vessels)
- Decreases inflammation
- Decreases blood clotting (antagonist of platelet-aggregating factor)
- Enhances learning and memorization
- Improves mood
- Helps prevent loss of memory
- Increases uptake of glucose
- Increases serotonin receptors
- Increases acetyl choline synthesis

Ginkgo is effective for treating the following:[2, 3, 4, 5, 6, 7, 8, 9]

- Memory loss
- Depression
- Peripherial vascular disease/claudication/pain in legs due to decreased circulation
- Impotence
- Macular degeneration

- Glaucoma
- Diabetic retinopathy
- Tinnitus (ringing in ears)
- Raynaud's disease

Dosage: 40-80 mg

Side effects: Ginkgo is a blood thinner. *If you are on blood thinners or are pregnant do not take ginkgo.*

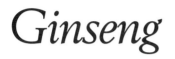

Ginseng

Asian Ginseng (Panax ginseng)

Asian ginseng does the following:[1]

- Helps relieve stress and anxiety
- Helps relieve insomnia and restlessness
- Is an adaptogen
- Relieves lethargy and fatigue
- Helps with forgetfulness
- Decreases bloating and fullness
- Increases energy
- Supports adrenal glands
- Decreases depression
- Improves mood
- Helps increase physical endurance
- Increases mental abilities
- Stimulates immune function
- Enhances heart function
- Helps with glucose metabolism

Dosage: 125-500 mg

Side effects: You may not be able to take Asian ginseng if you have anxiety or insomnia.

Siberian Ginseng
(Eleutherococcus senticosus)

Siberian ginseng does the following:[2]

- Aids the immune system (increases T cell and natural killer cell activity)
- Acts as an adaptogen
- Increases physical performance and stamina
- Increases mental awareness
- Improves learning ability
- Promotes healing
- Acts as a stimulant
- Helps you deal with stress
- Increases tolerance to excess noise, heat, and workload

Dosage: 500-1,000 mg

Glutathione

12

Glutathione is composed of three amino acids: glycine, glutamic acid, and cysteine. After the age of 40, the production of glutathione by your body diminishes.

Functions of glutathione:[1]

- Is the "master antioxidant"
- Is a neurotransmitter
- Is a neuromodulator
- Displaces glutamate from its binding site
- Helps to recycle other antioxidants such as vitamins C and E
- Regulates immune cells by stimulating interleukin 1 and 2 production
- Enhances liver and brain detoxification of toxic chemicals and heavy metals
- Used in DNA synthesis and repair
- Involved in protein and prostaglandin synthesis
- Part of amino acid transport
- Decreases your craving for sugar

Nutrients that can boost glutathione in your body:[2, 3]

- Vitamin C
- Alpha lipoic acid
- Glutamine
- Methionine
- S-adenosyl methionine (SAMe)
- Whey protein
- Vitamin E
- Milk thistle

Things that decrease glutathione:[4]

- Cigarette smoking
- Overly processed chemical-laden foods such as luncheon meats that contain nitrites or nitrates
- Excessive intake of alcohol
- Acetaminophen

Glutathione is not effective if taken by mouth because it is broken down by digestive enzymes. It can be taken, however, as a specific form of amino acid linkage that is not broken down by digestive enzymes called n-acetylcysteine (NAC).

Natural sources of glutathione can be found in asparagus, avocado, walnuts, fish, and meat.

Dosage: 500-3,000 mg of NAC. Glutathione can also be given by your physician as an IV.

Side effects: *NAC should be used only with extra vitamin C in order to avoid kidney stone formation.* Cysteine can precipitate and cause kidney stones. *Also, if you are taking NAC for prolonged periods of time then you may need to take extra copper and zinc since NAC can bind these minerals and make them unavailable for usage in your body.*

13

Hawthorn
(Crataegus laevigata)

Hawthorn contains procyanidins and the flavonoids rutin, quercetin, hyperoside, and vitexin.

Functions of hawthorn:[1]
- Normalizes blood pressure
- Prevents heart racing
- Keeps heart rhythm regular
- Dilates blood vessels and improves blood low
- Stabilizes collagen
- Is an antioxidant

Hawthorn is used in the treatment of:[2]
- High blood pressure
- Coronary heart disease
- Congestive heart failure
- Arthritis

Indole-3-Carbinol (I-3-C)

14

Helps prevent the development of estrogen-enhanced cancers including breast, uterine, and cervical.[1,2,3,4] Indole-3-carbinol has protective affects on the prostate as well.[5]

Foods that contain indole-3-carbinol include: broccoli, Brussels sprouts, kale, and cabbage.

Dosage: 300-500 mg

Alpha Lipoic Acid 15

Alpha lipoic acid is a nutrient that is both fat and water-soluble. As you age your body makes less alpha lipoic acid.

Functions of alpha lipoic acid:[1, 2, 3, 4, 5, 6, 7, 8, 9]

- Is a cofactor of mitochondrial enzymes needed for energy production
- Helps insulin work more effectively
- Improves your immune system
- Protects collagen in the skin from cross-linking and causing wrinkles
- Acts as a metal chelator for iron, copper, and cadmium
- Recycles vitamins E, C, glutathione, and coenzyme Q-10
- Helps prevent cataracts
- Lowers levels of copper and calcium if you have too much
- Stimulates the sprouting of new nerve fibers on nerve cells
- Stops the adhesion of macrophages to your artery wall (helps prevent heart disease)
- Stops NF kappa B activation in your cells which leads to heart disease
- Increases glutathione by 30 to 70 percent
- Modulates gene expression
- Strengthens memory and prevents brain aging

It is impossible to eat enough lipoic acid to be therapeutic. You would have to eat 100 pounds of spinach to equal a 100 mg capsule of lipoic acid.[10]

Alpha lipoic acid is used in the treatment of:[11, 12, 13, 14, 15]

- Diabetes mellitus
- Hepatitis C
- Maintain memory
- AIDS
- Psoriasis
- Eczema
- Burns
- Skin cancer
- Immunosuppression
- Multiple sclerosis
- Lou Gehrig's disease
- Parkinson's disease
- Rheumatoid arthritis
- Lupus
- Scleroderma
- Macular degeneration
- Cataracts
- Heart disease
- Circulatory disorders
- Stroke
- Atherosclerosis
- Diabetic neuropathy

Melatonin

16

Melatonin is a hormone. The amount of melatonin your body produces depends on the activity of an enzyme called serotonin-N-acetyl-transferase (NAT). Vitamin B6 is needed for NAT.

Functions of melatonin in your body:[1, 2, 3]
- Helps you get to sleep and stay asleep
- Decreases your risk of heart disease by decreasing atherosclerosis
- Promotes healthy cholesterol levels
- Decreases platelet stickiness
- Strengthens the immune system
- Acts as an antioxidant

Causes of decreased melatonin levels:[4]
- Medications

Acetaminophen	Diltiazem
Alcohol	Filodipine
Aprazolam	Flunitrazepam
Aspirin	Fluoxetine
Atenolol	Ibuprofen
Benzerazide	Indomethacin
Bepridil	Interleukin-2
Clonidine	Isradapine
Dexamethasone	Luzindole
Diazepam	Methylcobalamine

Metoprolol	Nitrendipine
Nicardipine	Prazosin
Nifedipine	Propanolol
Nimodipine	Reserpine
Nisoldipine	Ridazolol

- Caffeine
- Tobacco
- Alcohol
- Vitamin B12

Causes of increased melatonin levels:[5]

- Taking melatonin as a supplement
- Medications such as thorazine, fluvoxamine, desipramine, clorgyline, tranylcypromine
- St. John's wort
- Foods such as oats, sweat corn, rice, ginger, tomatoes, bananas, and barley

New research is demonstrating that melatonin is very helpful in the treatment of breast cancer.[6, 7]

Side effects: *Melatonin is an immune stimulator. Consequently if you have an autoimmune disease you should not take it. Furthermore, you should not take melatonin if you are pregnant, on prescription steroids, have depression, mental illness, lymphoma, or leukemia.*

Dosage: *1-6 mg one hour before bedtime.*

17

Milk Thistle (Silymarin/ Silybum marianuum)

Extract from the seeds of the milk thistle plant contains silibinin which is a substance that helps keep you healthy.

Functions of milk thistle:[1, 2, 3, 4, 5, 6, 7]
- Protects your liver from damage due to toxins
- Increases production of glutathione
- Maintains bile flow
- Reduces inflammation
- Diminishes oxidation
- Increases growth of new tissue to repair damaged areas
- Helps prevent damage due to excessive alcohol ingestion
- Protects against iron damage in the liver
- Lowers cholesterol
- Increases HDL (good cholesterol)
- Decreases the oxidation of LDL (bad cholesterol)
- Decreases blood sugar
- Helps protect kidneys from the effects of cisplatin
- Is an antioxidant

Dosage:
- Diabetes   250 mg
- Increase glutathione   150-300 mg
- Liver disease   400-800 mg

MSM

18

(Methylsulfonylmethane)

MSM is a natural substance that you make in your body and is also present in certain foods. It is used to treat pain and inflammation. MSM supplies the mineral sulfur to your body. This is *not* sulfa. You *can* take MSM if you are allergic to sulfa.

MSM provides pain relief through the following ways:[1]
- The inhibition of pain impulses along nerve fibers
- Lessening of inflammation
- Increasing of blood supply
- Reduction of muscle spasm
- Softening of scar tissue
- Reduces muscle spasm
- Immune normalizing effect

MSM is used in the following conditions:[2]
- Osteoarthritis
- Rheumatoid arthritis
- Chronic back pain
- Chronic headaches
- Muscle pain
- Fibromyalgia
- Tendonitis and bursitis
- Carpal tunnel syndrome

- TMJ
- Inflammation after an injury
- Heartburn
- Allergies

Sulfur is a major ingredient of the amino acids methionine and cysteine. Sulfur is present naturally in cabbage, kale, kohlrabi, Brussels sprouts, mustard greens, watercress, leeks, onion, radish, cauliflower, and horseradish.[3]

Dosage: 2,000 to 10,000 mg

19

OPCs (Oligomeric Proanthocyanidin Complexes)

OPCs are flavonoids that are powerful antioxidants. Your body cannot make them. The richest sources of OPCs are found in red wine extract, grape seed extract, and pine bark extract.

Red wine extract:[1, 2]

- Prevents platelet stickiness
- Decreases cholesterol
- Reduces triglycerides
- Lowers apolipoprotein B
- Anticancer effects

Grape seed extract:[3, 4, 5]

- Lowers LDL (bad) cholesterol
- Anticancer effects
- Is an antioxidant
- Prevents damage to DNA
- Increases immune system

Pine bark:[6]

- Protects your cells from oxidative damage
- Helps treat venous insufficiency
- Boost immune system
- Anticancer effects

OPCs are used to treat:[7]

- Chronic fatigue syndrome
- Arthritis
- High cholesterol
- Alzheimer's disease

20

Phosphatidyl choline (Lecithin)

Phosphatidyl choline is used in the treatment of:[1, 2, 3]
- High homocysteine
- Decreased liver function
- Fibrocystic breast disease
- Fibroids
- Memory loss
- Helps convert estradiol (E2) to estriol (E3)

Dosage: 1-20 grams.

Alpha-GPC
(Alpha-Glyceryl phosphoryl choline)

Alpha-GPC is a derivative of soy lecithin that contains choline. It is a direct precursor in the making of choline in your body. Choline makes acetylcholine, which is a neurotransmitter involved with communication in your brain.

Acetyl choline sensitive neurons have the following functions:[4]
- Control of arousal
- Learning and memory
- Motor activity
- REM sleep
- May increase growth hormone release

Taking alpha-GPC is preferred over choline or lecithin since it allows for a greater amount of choline to be absorbed by your gut.

Dosage: 100-500 mg

Phosphatidylserine 21

Phosphatidylserine is a phospholipid. Phospho means it contains phosphorus and lipid means it contains fat molecules. It is in a complex with the amino acid serine. Phosphatidylserine is one of the key building blocks in your brain. It is also present in all cells in your body.

Functions of phosphatidylserine in your body:[1, 2, 3]

- Reduces cortisol (stress hormone)
- Influences the fluidity of nerve-cell membranes
- Needed for electrical activity of the brain
- Incorporates membrane proteins
- Critical for neurotransmission
- Used in bone matrix formation
- Testicular function
- Heart rhythm
- Immune function

Phosphatidylserine is used in the treatment of:[4, 5, 6, 7, 8, 9, 10, 11, 12]

- Memory decline including Alzheimer's disease
- Anxiety
- Depression
- Motor function in Parkinson's disease
- Improving learning, concentration, and work skills
- Stress

Side effects: None.

Dosage: 100-500 mg

22

Probiotics

Probiotics are the friendly bacteria in your intestines that increase your defenses against disease.

Functions of probiotics in your body:

- Plays a major role in digestion
- Helps manufacture niacin, folic acid, and biotin
- Makes lactase, an enzyme needed to help the digestion of milk products
- Increases your immune system (increases white blood cells, increases phagocytosis, increases gama-interferon)

Over use of antibiotics and poor nutritional intake can create an overgrowth in your bowel of unhealthy bacteria. The probiotics mentioned in this book that are used in our office are called Ultra Flora Plus made by Metagenics (see Appendix for availability).

23

Pycnogenol

Pycogenol is the name that is trademarked for a mixture of forty different antioxidants that are from the bark of the pine tree (Pinus maritime).

Functions of pycogenol:[1]

- Increases the life time of vitamin C in your body
- Can elevate your body's production of vitamin E and glutathione
- Improves the circulation in your capillaries
- Protects against platelet stickiness
- Stimulates natural killer cells that help your body fight off cancer
- Relieves inflammation
- Helps regulate nitric oxide production

Resveratrol

24

Resveratrol is a polyphenol (bioflavonoid) in wine, grapes, peanuts, and mulberries.

Functions of resveratrol:[1, 2, 3, 4, 5, 6, 7, 8, 9]
- Is an anti-inflammatory
- Induces phase II detoxification enzymes
- Inhibits COX-2 enzyme induction
- Decreases lipooxygenase
- Opens arteries by increasing nitric oxide
- Inhibits mitochondrial ROS formation
- Inhibits LDL (bad cholesterol) oxidation
- Decreases platelet stickiness
- Helps prevent cancer
- Stops the proliferation of cells that narrow your arteries
- Helps prevent Alzheimer's disease
- Is an antioxidant

Dosage: 20 mg. In our office we use resveratrol from Life Extensions (see Appendix for availability).

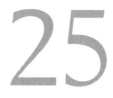

Saw Palmetto
(Serenoa repens)

Saw palmetto is an herb that is used to treat an enlarged prostate gland.[1] It can also lower testosterone in women with excess levels of this hormone.[2]

Dosage:
- 160 mg is the average dose for an enlarged prostate.
- 500 mg is used to lower testosterone in women.

26

Vinpocetine

Vinpocetine is from the periwinkle plant.

Functions of vinpocetine:[1]
- Increases memory in the following ways:
  Increases blood flow
  Increases the rate at which your brain cells produce ATP (create energy)
  Speeds up the use of glucose in your brain (its main fuel source)
  Improves the utilization of oxygen by your brain
- Inhibits platelet aggregation (stickiness)
- Decreases the deformity of RBC (red blood cells)
- Increases serotonin
- Helps with hair loss

Vinpocetine is used in the treatment of the following:[2, 3, 4]
- Stroke
- Vertigo
- Meniere's Syndrome
- Sleep disorders
- Mood changes
- Depression
- Tinnitis (ringing in ears)
- Sensorineural hearing loss
- Migraine headaches
- Macular degeneration
- Seizure disorder
- Headache

Dosage: 10-40 mg

27

Juice Plus

Juice Plus is a nutraceutical that provides whole food based nutrition from 17 different fruits, vegetables, and grains plus fiber blends and acidophilus in the form of a capsule, chewable tablet, or gummie. Apples, oranges, pineapples, cranberries, peaches, cherries, papaya, carrots, spinach, broccoli, kale, cabbage, parsley, beets, and tomato are all included in Juice Plus.

Research has shown that Juice Plus supplementation does the following:[1, 2, 3]

- Significantly raises the levels of key antioxidants in the blood stream
- Improves major immune functions
- Reduces DNA damage
- Significantly improves blood circulation following a high-fat meal
- Reduces serum homocysteine levels

I use Juice Plus in my office. For a Juice Plus representative near you see the Appendix.

The treatment of disease is a matter of varying the concentration of substances (i.e., the right molecules: vitamins, minerals, trace elements, hormones, amino acids, enzymes) normally present in the body.
—Linus Pauling, Ph.D.

Section 7
Nutritional Programs

This section of the book includes selected suggested programs for prevention, maintaining optimal health, and specific diseases. They are by no means comprehensive. The dosages are set for adults and for people without kidney or liver disease except where indicated. *If you have kidney or liver disease, dosages may need to be lowered. If you are pregnant or nursing, consult your doctor before following any of these protocols.*

For many of these chapters a number of different therapeutic options are listed and they do not all have to be used simultaneously. Some of the suggested nutrients are based on published medical research. Other programs are based on clinical observations by the doctors at The Center For Healthy Living, as well as other physician's usage, and from medical conferences attended.

This section is not designed to be a cookbook for nutritional treatment of disease or a cookbook on how to maintain optimal health. *Treatment should be individualized. One size does not fit all!* As always, working with a health professional trained in nutrition and functional medicine is suggested. For a list of how to find a functional medicine or anti-aging healthcare provider please refer to the introduction of this book.

Wherever MVI is listed this stands for multi-vitamin.

If you are taking coumadin or any other blood thinner then your dosage of vitamin E, garlic, and ginkgo must be lower than what is suggested in the following programs. Please contact your physician as to the appropriate dosage change.

If you are having surgery then do not take any of these nutrients (except for the surgery pre and post operative protocol) two weeks before and after your date of surgery.

ADD /ADHD

1

ADD/ADHD can be inherited. The cause may also be due to brain injury, toxic exposure, or high fever.[1] Food allergies, metal toxicities, EPA/DHA deficiencies (pre-natally), diet, zinc deficiencies, and zinc/copper imbalance also play a role.[2]

The goal of a functional treatment for ADD/ADHD is not only to improve performance on repetitive tasks but also to expand academic skills. Research shows that medications will not expand academic skill learning.[3] Furthermore, stimulant medications and amphetamines traditionally used to treat ADD/ADHD reduce the overall blood flow to the brain, disturb glucose metabolism, and may cause permanent shrinkage or atrophy to the brain according to Peter Breggin M.D. in his book entitled *Talking Back to Ritalin.*[4] Consequently, we use a functional approach to treatment of ADD/ADHD by testing for food allergies, toxic metals, and nutritional therapies that have been shown to be medically affective.

Supplements:[5, 6, 7, 8, 9, 10, 11, 12, 13, 14, 15]

EPA/DHA	500-1,000 mg
Magnesium	250-500 mg
Carnitine	4,000 mg
Zinc	25-50 mg
American ginseng	200 mg
Ginkgo	60 mg twice a day

St. John's wort	300-1200 mg (cannot take if on an anti-depressant)
Phosphatidylserine	100-500 mg
GLA	240-720 mg
B complex vitamins	50-100 mg
Selenium	100 micrograms
Boron	5-10 mg
Probiotics	Ultra flora plus
B12	500-1,000 micrograms
Folic acid	500-1,000 micrograms
5-HTP	100-200 mg
L-carnitine	1,000-2,000 mg

Also avoid sugar, food additives, and colorings.

Allergies

2

Food allergies are very common. Scientists estimate that 60% of the U.S. population suffers from food reactions.[1] Some are immediate which means they occur within three hours after eating the offending food. Delayed reactions can occur even days after eating the food you are allergic to. Eliminate the allergy creating item. *You might actually crave the exact food you are allergic to.*

Symptoms of food allergies:[2]

- Tension headaches
- Itchy, watery eyes
- Red eyes
- Anal itching
- Fluid behind eardrum
- Ringing in ears
- Hearing loss
- Red rosy cheeks
- Red earlobes
- Dark circles under eyes
- Wrinkles under eyes
- Cracks at corners of mouth
- Hoarseness
- Rapid heart beat
- Heart palpitations
- Belching
- Heartburn
- Indigestion
- Stomach aches
- Spastic colon
- Diarrhea
- Hives
- Eczema
- Muscle cramps
- Backaches
- Frequency and burning with urination
- Anemia
- Sluggishness
- Depression
- Restlessness
- Nervousness
- Tremors
- Emotional outbursts

- Destructive behavior
- Anxiety, fear
- Phobias, panic attacks
- Spacey feeling
- Memory loss
- Inability to concentrate
- Irritable behavior after meals

Supplements:[3, 4, 5, 6, 7, 8, 9, 10]

Perilla seed extract	Metagenics *(see Appendix for availability)*
EPA/DHA	1,000-2,000 mg
Vitamin C	1,000-2,000 mg
Probiotics	Ultra flora plus
GLA	240 mg 1 to 3 times a day
Quercetin	500-1,000 mg
Magnesium	400-600 mg
B vitamin complex	100 mg
Selenium	200-400 micrograms
Vitamin E	400-800 IU
Zinc	25 mg
Glutamine	1-10 grams
Curcumin	100-1,000 mg
Alpha lipoic acid	200-300 mg

Alzheimer's Disease 3

Supplements:[1, 2, 3, 4, 5, 6, 7, 8, 9, 10, 11, 12, 13, 14, 15, 16, 17, 18, 19, 20, 21, 22, 23, 24, 25, 26, 27]

Acetyl-L-carnitine	1,500-3,000 mg
Phosphatidylserine	300-500 mg
Vitamin E	400-2,000 IU (mixed tocopherols)
Folic acid	1,000 micrograms
Vitamin B12	5,000-10,000 micrograms
Alpha-lipoic acid	200-400 mg
Phosphatidyl choline	200-600 mg
Gingkgo biloba	120-240 mg
Carotinoids	10,000-25,000 IU (8,000 IU if a smoker)
B complex	100 mg
Vitamin C	2,000-5,000 mg
Magnesium	400-600 mg
Selenium	200-400 micrograms
Coenzyme Q-10	100-300 mg
NADH	10 mg
NAC	2,000 mg
Inositol	5,000-10,000 mg
Bilberry	200 mg
Huperzine A	50 micrograms
Vitamin D	600-800 IU
EPA/DHA	1,000-2,000 mg
Vinpocetine	10-40 mg

4

Anorexia

Supplements:[1]

Zinc	25-50 mg
Flax seed oil	1 tablespoon
GLA	480-720 mg
MVI	
Vitamin A	5,000 IU
L-taurine	500 mg
Magnesium	400 mg
Amino acid supplements	(individualized using amino acid testing)
EPA/DHA	500 mg
Carnitine	500 mg
Coenzyme Q-10	30 mg

5

Anxiety

Anxiety is a common problem with as many as 10 million Americans suffering from anxiety or panic attacks.[1]

Supplements:[2, 3]

Calcium	600-1,200 mg
Magnesium	300-600 mg
B complex	100 mg
Inositol	12 grams
GABA	375-750 mg three times a day
Glutamine	1,000 mg
Glycine	1,000 mg

Avoid sugar, caffeine, and alcohol.

6

Arthritis

The key to treating osteoarthritis is to decrease inflammation. Rheumatoid arthritis, has an inflammatory component that requires treatment along with the need to stabilize the immune system.

The following nutrients will all work for inflammation. They are grouped according to classifications.

Agents to decrease inflammation:[1]
- Essential fatty acids
  EPA
  GLA
- Niacinamide
- Pantothenic acid
- Proteases (bromelain)
- Glucosamine
- Bioflavonoids
  Quercitin
  Grape seed extract
  Hesperidin
- Antioxidants

Plant pigments with antioxidant properties:[2]
- Carotenoids (lycopene, beta carotene)
- Green tea catechins (polyphenols)
- Anthocyanidins (beets, berries, grapes)

- Quercitin (fruits and vegetable rind)
- Curcuminoids (tumeric)
- Trans-resveratrol (a phytoalexin from grapes)

Potent herbal antioxidants:[3]
- Ashwaganda (Withania somnifera)
- Blueberry/bilberry (Vaccinium myrtillus)
- Chocolate (Theobroma cacao)
- Cranberry (Vaccinium macrocarpon)
- Garlic (Allium sativum)
- Gingko (Gingko biloba)
- Ginger (Zingiber officinalis)
- Green tea (Camellia sinensis)
- Grape seed (Vitus vinifera)
- Hawthorn (Crataegus oxyacantha)
- Horse chestnut (Aesculus hippocastanum)
- Milk thistle (Silybum marianum)
- Oregano (Origanum vulgare)
- Purple grape (Vitis labrusca)
- Rosemary (Rosmarinus officinalis)
- Turmeric (Curcuma longa)

Botanicals found to have anti-inflammatory properties:[4]
- Willow bark (Salix species)
- Licorice root (Glycyrrhiza glabra)
- Boswellia (Boswellia serrata)
- Bromelain (Ananus comosus)
- Chinese skullcap (Scutellaria baicalensis)
- Turmeric (Curcuma longa)
- Ginger (Zingiber officinalis) *Do take with coumadin or non-steroidal anti-inflammatory medications.*
- Cayenne pepper (Capsicum annuum)
- Aloe vera (Aloe barbadensis)
- Green tea (Camellia sinensis)
- Ginkgo (Ginkgo biloba)

Natural COX-2 inhibitors:[5]
- Bromelain (Pineapple stem: Ananus comosus)
- Capsaicin (Cayenne: Capsicum annuum)
- Carnosol and carnosic acid (Rosemary)
- Carvacrol (Oregano: Origanum vulgare)
- Chinese skullcap (Scutellaria baicalensis)
- Curcumin (Turmeric: Curcuma longa) *Do not take with non-steroidal anti-inflammatory medications.*
- Feverfew (Tanacetum parthenium)
- Gamma tocopherol
- Gingerol/Shogaol (Ginger: Zingiber officinalis)
- Green tea catechins (Camellia sinensis)
- Melatonin (Ginger, Seaweed)
- Trans-resveratrol (Purple grape)
- Thymol (Thyme: Thymus bulgaris)
- Quercitin
- Willow bark (Salix species)

Osteoarthritis
Supplements:[6, 7, 8, 9, 10, 11, 12, 13, 14, 15]

MSM	1,000-6,000 mg
Chondroitin sulfate	300-2,000 mg
Boron	1,000 micrograms
B complex vitamins	50-100 mg
EPA/DHA	1,000-2,000 mg
Glucosamine sulfate	1,500-3,000 mg
Kaprex	2-4 tablets (made by Metagenics)
Ultrainflammax (a medical food product with anti-inflammatory botanicals made by Metagenics)	2 scoops twice a day
Quercetin	500-1,000 mg
GLA	240-720 mg
Manganese	5-10 mg
Ginger	100 mg

Rheumatoid Arthritis

Supplements:[16, 17, 18, 19, 20, 21, 22, 23]

Zinc	25 mg
B complex vitamins	100 mg
Magnesium	600 mg
EPA/DHA	1,500-2,000 mg
L-arginine	2,000 mg
Glutamine	1,500 mg
NAC	500-1,000 mg
Coenzyme Q-10	60-120 mg
L-carnitine	500-1,000 mg
Vitamin C	1,000-2,000 mg
Lipoic acid	300-600 mg
Ginger	100 mg
GLA	900 mg
Curcumin	100-1,000 mg
Bioflavanoids	
Selenium	100-200 micrograms
MSM	3,000-10,000 mg
Tumeric rhizome	300 mg
Boswellia resin	400 mg
Copper	2 mg

Patients with rheumatoid arthritis should decrease their intake of foods from the night shade group including tomatoes, potatoes, and eggplants.

Gout

Supplements:[24]

Folic acid	10-20 mg
Alpha lipoic acid	2, 000 mg
EPA/DHA	2,000 mg
Carnitine	1,000 amg
Coenzyme Q-10	120 mg

Milk thistle	300 mg
Chromium	400-1,000 micrograms
Vitamin C	1,000-3,000 mg
Vitamin E	400 IU
Quercetin	500 mg
Chamomile (Matricaria recutita)	3 capsules or 3 cups of tea
Yarrow (Achillea millefolium)	3 capsules
Baikal skullcap (Scuttelaria baicalensis)	3 capsules
Bilberry	60 mg
Grape seed extract	300-900 mg
Celery seed extract	450 mg

Avoid niacin in B complex vitamins since it competes with uric acid for excretion and it will make the gouty attack worse. Avoid organ meats, anchovies, baker's and brewer's yeast, herring, mackerel, red meat, sardines, shellfish, game meat, high fructose corn syrup, vitamin A, high dose molybdenum (1,000 micrograms or more a day).

7

Asthma

Supplements:[1, 2, 3, 4, 5, 6, 7]

EPA/DHA	2,000 mg
Magnesium	400-600 mg
MSM	3,000-15,000 mg
Vitamin B12	5,000 micrograms
Vitamin C	2,000 mg
B complex	100 mg
Folic acid	1,000 mg
Selenium	400 micrograms
Carotenoids	50-5,000 IU
	(consult physician doses greater than 10,000)
Vitamin E	400-800 IU
Zinc	25 mg
Probiotics	Ultra flora plus
Curcumin	100-1,000 mg
Quercetin	300-900 mg
Taurine	1,000-3,000 mg
NAC	1,000-2,000 mg
Grape seed extract	300 mg three times a day
Gingko biloba	80-240 mg

8

Autoimmune Diseases—To Quiet Your Immune Response

An autoimmune disease process is a state where your immune system is functioning too much, called hyper-immune function.

Symptoms of hyper-immune function:[1]
- Muscles fatigue quickly
- Moody, irritable, tired
- Severe fatigue
- Severe joint pain, redness, swelling
- Pain, stiffness throughout your body
- Migraine headaches
- Sensitive to light (skin or eyes)
- Dark circles under eyes
- Swollen-looking face or body
- Localized or general itching
- Clear, watery discharge from nose, eyes
- Extreme dryness of eyes, nasal passages, mouth
- Sneezing
- Cough or wheezing
- Postnasal drip with certain foods

- Heart palpitations after eating particular foods
- Weight loss
- Muscle weakness
- Loss of hair (head and rest of body)
- Easy bruising
- Nails loosened, pitted, discolored
- Foot pain, inflammation, stiffness
- Moldy, damp environments trigger sickness

The following protocols can be used for Crohn's disease, Hashimoto's thyroiditis, lupus, myasthenia gravis, rheumatoid arthritis, and Sjogren's syndrome.

Supplements:[2, 3, 4, 5]

EPA/DHA	1,000-5,000 mg
	(may use up to 10,000 under physician direction)
Glutamine	1-5 grams
GLA	240-720 mg
Flaxseed	1,000 mg
Vitamin C	1,000-3,000 mg
Vitamin E	400 IU
Selenium	200-400 micrograms
Magnesium	400-800 mg
Siberian ginseng	50-200 mg
Olive leaf extract	1-3 capsules
Probiotics	Ultra flora plus
Glucosamine	300-900 mg

Scleroderma (Systemic Sclerosis)

Supplements:[6, 7, 8]

PABA	3-12 grams
Probiotics	Ultra flora plus
EPA/DHA	1,000-4,000 mg
Glutamine	1,000-10,000 mg
GLA	240-720 mg

Flax seed oil	1-3 tablespoons
Vitamin C	1,000-5,000 mg
Vitamin E	400-800 IU
	(lower doses are needed if on a blood thinner)
Selenium	200 micrograms
Carnitine	1,000-2,000 mg
Glucosamine	300-900 mg

Do not fear cancer. The human body is incredibly
tough. Given the right nutrition, exercise, and
lifestyle, it will resist cancer for a lifetime.

9

—Professor Lewis Thomas, President of
Sloan Kettering Cancer Hospital

Cancer

An article published in a recent cancer journal posed the question: Are vitamin and mineral deficiencies a major cancer risk? Dr. Bruce Ames, author of the article, stated that "diet is expected to contribute to about one third of preventable cancers—about the same as cigarette smoking . . . Recent experimental evidence indicates that vitamin and mineral differences can lead to DNA damage. Optimizing vitamin and mineral intake by encouraging dietary change, multivitamin and mineral supplements, and fortifying foods might therefore prevent cancer and other chronic disease."

Supplements: [1, 2, 3, 4, 5, 6, 7, 8, 9, 10, 11, 12, 13, 14, 15, 16, 17, 18, 19, 20]

Vitamin A	5,000 IU
Mixed carotenoids	5,000 IU
Lycopene	10-20 mg
Vitamin C	1,000-2,000 mg
Vitamin E	400 IU
Niacinamide	100-1,000 mg
Tocotrienols	100-200 mg
Vitamin D	400-800 IU
Magnesium	600 mg
Zinc	25 mg
Selenium	100-200 micrograms
Iodine	150 micrograms

Flax seed	1,000 mg
Coenzyme Q-10	100-400 mg
	(400 mg in breast cancer) *divided*
CLA	100-300 mg
Lipoic acid	100-300 mg
Chlorella	1 tablespoon
Quercetin	300-900 mg
I-3-C (indole-3-carbinol)	300-500 mg – *divided*
Folic acid	100-800 micrograms
Pycnogenol	20 mg
Melatonin	1-20 mg *Start with 1 mg @ bedtime and ↑ if no side effects*
Curcumin	100-1,000 mg

+ Omega 3's (EPA/DHA) 2-3 gms/day – divided

+ green tea – 3 cups/day or take supplement

+ SAME

10

Candidiasis (Yeast Infections) and Dysbiosis

Candida albicans is a yeast that invades your mouth, throat, intestines, urinary and genital areas. It is a normal part of your gut flora but can, under certain conditions, grow uncontrolled. Infections by yeast contribute to a condition called candida-related complex.

Causes of candidiasis:
- Chronic antibiotic use
- Oral birth control
- Excess sugar intake
- Diabetes
- Decreased immune system

Major symptoms of candida-related complex:[1]
- Fatigue
- Poor memory
- Feeling "spacey" or "unreal"
- Bloating, intestinal gas
- Vaginal itching, burning, discharge
- Numbness, burning, tingling
- Insomnia
- Muscle aches, weakness
- Abdominal pain
- Constipation
- Prostatitis
- PMS
- Anxiety/crying
- Shaking or irritability when hungry

Other symptoms:[2]

- Headaches
- Sinusitis
- Moodiness
- White tongue
- Tendency to bruise easily
- Chronic rashes, itching
- Food sensitivity or intolerance
- Mucus in stools
- Rectal itching
- Hoarseness, loss of voice
- Nasal itching

To test for a yeast infection our office uses a CDSA test from Great Smokies Laboratory (see Appendix for availability).

Treatment:[3]

- Prescription anti-fungal agent e.g., nystatin, diflucan
- Red thyme oil
- Oregano leaf extract
- Sage leaf
- Coptis root
- Rhizome extract
- Barberry root
- Berberine sulfate
- Garlic
- Grape seed extract
- Black walnut hull
- Slippery elm bark
- Goldenseal root
- Bearberry leaf
- Caprylic acid
- Undecyclenic acid
- Plant tannins: acerin, quebracho, lotus rhizome, Swedish birch bark, babul bark
- Berberine: hydrastis (golden seal), berberis (Oregon grape root), echinacea
- Oregano oil
- Uva ursi
- Paud arco

- Biocidin
- Glutamine   5-10 grams per day
- Zinc   25 mg
- B complex vitamins 50-100 mg
- Arginine   1-5 grams
- Molybdenum   250-500 micrograms

In my office we use CandiBactin-AR and CandiBactin BR made by Metagenics (for availability see the Appendix). CandiBactin-AR contains red thyme oil, oregano leaf extract, sage leaf, and lemon balm leaf. Candibactin-BR contains coptis root, rhizome extract, barberry root extract, and berberine sulfate.

Be aware, that your symptoms may get worse for a week or two as the yeast die off and again in 21 days as the budding yeast expire. It is also helpful to take probiotics (beneficial bacteria).

After two months, you can stop the glutamine and continue the good bacteria twice a week.

Nutrients helpful in long term management of yeast overgrowth:

Carnitine	1,000-3,000 mg
Vitamin C	1,000 mg
Vitamin E	400 IU
Magnesium	400-800 mg
Chromium	300 micrograms
Taurine	1-3 grams
GLA	240-480 mg

11

Nutrients That Are Good For Your Heart

These nutrients help prevent atherosclerosis which is a build up of fat deposits on the walls of your arteries.

Supplements:[1, 2, 3, 4, 5, 6, 7, 8, 9]

Niacin	100 mg
Chromium	400 micrograms
Carnitine	1,000-4,000 mg
Vitamin C	1,000-5,000 mg
Vitamin E	400-800 IU
B complex	100 mg
Folic acid	500 micrograms
Vitamin B12	500-1,000 micrograms
Coenzyme Q-10	60-100 mg
Copper	2-4 mg
Zinc	25-50 mg
Taurine	1,000-2,000 mg
Lecithin	2,000-4,000 mg
GLA	480 mg
Fiber (soluble)	Metafiber by Metagenics (see Appendix)
Magnesium	500-1,000 mg
EPA/DHA	500-2,000 mg

11.1 Cholesterol Lowering

There are many ways to lower cholesterol without using prescription medications. This chapter will look at how to lower total cholesterol, how to lower LDL (bad) cholesterol, how to lower triglycerides, how to raise HDL (good) cholesterol, and how to decrease platelet stickiness. It will also look at reasons for high and low cholesterol.

LDL cholesterol transports cholesterol to your various organs. HDL cholesterol transports excess cholesterol to the liver for breakdown and elimination from your body. You can keep your LDL (bad) cholesterol very low and your HDL (good) cholesterol very high, but if your LDL cholesterol oxidizes you will still develop heart disease (atherosclerosis). Cells called macrophages in your artery walls recognize the oxidized LDL as toxic to your body and attack them. If you have too many LDLs, the macrophages become fat and break down into cells, called foam cells, that form the fatty streaks on the walls of your arteries and are the beginning of atherosclerosis. Vitamin C prevents macrophages from absorbing LDL to begin with.[1]

One half of people who die of a heart attack have a normal cholesterol. Sections 11.2-11.6 of this chapter look at other risk factors for heart disease such as elevated homocysteine, high lipoprotein (a), increased fibrinogen, high c-reactive protein, and excess iron levels.

Causes of high cholesterol:[2]
- Excess dietary sugar
- Excess dietary starch
- Hydrogenated, partially hydrogenated, or processed fats (lard, shortening, cottonseed oil, palm oil, margarine)
- Liver dysfunction
- Amino acid deficiency
- Essential fatty acid deficiency
- Deficiency of natural antioxidants such as vitamin E, selenium, beta-carotene

- Increased tissue damage due to infection, radiation, or oxidative activity (free radical production)
- Fiber deficiency
- Vitamin C deficiency
- Carnitine deficiency
- Biotin deficiency
- Food allergies
- Alcoholism
- Hormone deficiency (testosterone, DHEA, estrogen)

If your cholesterol is too low (below 140), you cannot make your sex hormones at a normal level (DHEA, estrogen, progesterone, testosterone, and pregnenolone).

Causes of low cholesterol levels:[3]

- Immune decline
- Chronic hepatitis
- Cholesterol lowering drugs
- Essential fatty acid deficiency
- Liver infection or disease
- Manganese deficiency
- Adrenal stress
- Recreational drugs (cocaine, marijuana)
- Excessive exercise (especially in females)
- Low fat diets
- Psychological stress
- Cancer

How to lower cholesterol:

- Policosanol[4, 5, 6, 7, 8, 9, 10, 11, 12, 13, 14, 15, 16]

   Made from sugar cane (diabetics may use)

   Blocks the synthesis of cholesterol

   Inhibits oxidation of LDL (bad) cholesterol

   Decreases platelet stickiness

   Raises HDL (good) cholesterol

   Dosage: 20 mg. In our office we use Cholarest made by Metagenics or policosanol made by Designs for Health or Life Extensions.

- Guggulipid (commiphora mukul)[17, 18, 19, 20, 21]

  Lowers LDL cholesterol

  Raises HDL cholesterol

  Lowers triglycerides

  Reduces platelet stickiness

  Acts as an antioxidant

  Dosage: 50 mg twice a day. In our office we use Lipotain made by Metagenics or policosanol + gugulipid made by Designs for Health.

- Tocotrienols (a special vitamin E)[22, 23]

  Modifies the expression and activity of HMGCoA reductase (this enzyme decreases how quickly your body makes cholesterol)

  Reduces apolipoprotein B and lipoprotein plasma levels

  Decreases plaque formation in your arteries

  Dosage: In our office we use Ultratrienols from Designs for Health.

- Garlic[24, 25]

  Decreases triglycerides

  Decreases total cholesterol

- Niacin[26]

  Decreases total cholesterol

  Decreases LDL

  Decreased triglycerides

  Increases HDL

  Side effects:

  Short term: flushing, itching, gut disturbances, weakness
  Long term: liver toxicity, high uric acid levels, glucose intolerance, eye disturbances, ulcers, postural hypotension

- Pantethine[27, 28, 29, 30, 31, 32]

  Decreases total cholesterol

  Decreases LDL

  Increases HDL

- Inositol[33]
  - ~~Decreases total cholesterol~~
  - Decreases LDL
  - Decreases triglycerides
  - Increases HDL
- Red Yeast Rice[34]
  - Decreases total cholesterol
  - Contains HMG-Co-A reductase inhibitors
  - *The active ingredient is now being taken out of some of the new red yeast rice products.*
- Fiber[35, 36, 37, 38]
  - Soluble fiber will lower both total and LDL cholesterol
- Exercise[39]
- Chromium[40, 41]
- Magnesium[42]
  - Decreases total cholesterol
  - Decreases LDL
  - Decreases triglycerides
  - Increases HDL
  - Decreases platelet stickiness
- Soy
  - Decreases total cholesterol
  - Decreases LDL
  - Decreases triglycerides
- L-carnitine[43]

11.2 Triglycerides

What causes triglycerides to rise?[1]

- White sugar
- White flour
- White bread, cakes, cookies, candies
- Soft drinks
- Alcohol
- Too much fruit
- Fruit juice
- High fat diet
- Family inheritance
- Skipping breakfast and/or lunch and making up for it at supper
- Lack of physical activity
- Stress
- Caffeine
- Nicotine
- Diuretics
- Birth control pills

How to lower triglycerides:[2, 3, 4, 5]

Decrease intake of fruits, no fruit juice

L-Carnitine	2,000 mg
EPA/DHA	1,000-2,000 mg
Chromium	300 micrograms
L-lysine	1,000 to 3000 mg
L-methionine	250-500 mg
Alpha ketoglutarate	500-1000 mg
L-arginine	2-4 grams
Magnesium	600-600 mg
Pantothenic acid	100 mg
Zinc	25 mg
Niacin	1-2 grams under the direction of a physician
Policosanol	10-20 mg

Guggulipid	500-1,000 mg
Tocotrienols	100-200 mg
Folic acid	2 mg
Vitamin B12	2,000 micrograms
Coenzyme Q-10	30-100 mg

Limit fruits and fruit juices.

Methods to increase HDL:

L-carnitine	1,000-2,000 mg
Niacin	100-1,000 mg
Guggulipid	100 mg
Policosanol	20 mg
Coenzyme Q-10	60-120 mg
Magnesium	600 mg
Pantethine	900 mg

11.3 Homocysteine

Homocysteine is an amino acid produced by ineffective protein metabolism that promotes free radical production.

Free radicals are molecules that lack an electron. They go searching in your body for an electron, will find a healthy cell, and steal an electron. This kills the cell. This is one of the causes of oxidative stress that leads to heart disease. Homocysteine also elevates triglycerides and cholesterol synthesis.[1]

Studies suggest that 42% of strokes, 28% of peripheral vascular disease (causes leg pain, cramping, and loss of circulation), and approximately 30% of cardiovascular disease (heart attacks, chest pain) are directly related to elevated homocysteine levels.[2, 3, 4] Furthermore, a study published in the New England Journal of Medicine in July 1997 showed that people with homocysteine levels below 9 were much less likely to die.[5] Another study showed that women with a history of high blood pressure and elevated homocysteine were 25 times more likely to have a heart attack or stroke.[6]

Homocysteine is increased in:[7, 8, 9, 10, 11]

- Coronary artery disease
- Dementia (memory loss)
- Diabetes
- Rheumatoid arthritis
- Osteoarthritis
- Menopause
- Hypothyroidism
- Drugs
- Toxins
- Smoking
- Renal failure
- Hereditary predisposition
- Elevated testosterone levels in women
- Memory loss

Ways to lower homocysteine:[12, 13, 14, 15, 16, 17, 18, 19, 20]

Vitamin B12	1,000 micrograms
Folic acid	800 micrograms
Vitamin B6	100 mg
Phosphatidyl choline	2,000-4,000 mg
Betaine (trimethylglycine)	500-1,000 mg
L-Taurine	2,000-4,000 mg
NAC	500-1,000 mg
Stop caffeine	
Stop diuretics	
Stop niacin	
Stop birth control pills	
Stop alcohol	
Stop tobacco	
MTHF (see below)	

Hereditary causes of high homocysteine may be due to the lack of an enzyme which breaks down homocysteine. It is called methylenetetrahydrofolate reductase.[21] A deficiency of this enzyme increases the need for folate in order to prevent a high homocysteine level. This occurs in 12% of the population.[22, 23, 24] In my practice I use the active form of folic acid (L-5-MTHF) for patients who take B6, B12, and folate but sill have elevated homocysteine levels. (For availability of this product, named FoloPro, see the Appendix under Metagenics.)

11.4 Fibrinogen

Fibrinogen is a clot-promoting substance in your blood. If the blood levels of fibrinogen are too high it can cause a heart attack.

Ways to lower fibrinogen:[1]
- Garlic
- EPA/DHA
- Vitamin E
- Ginger
- Bromelain
- Stop smoking
- Estrogen hormone replacement
- Ginkgo

11.5 Lipoprotein (a)

Lipoprotein (a) is a small cholesterol particle that causes inflammation and can clog your blood vessels.[1, 2] Research has shown that people with elevated lipoprotein (a) have a 70% higher risk of developing heart disease over 10 years.[3] Elevated lipoprotein (a) is inherited. Lipoprotein (a) regulates clot formation and decreases blood thinning.[4] This process is increased in diabetes and in menopause. *Also, statin medications (cholesterol lowering) have been shown to increase lipoprotein (a) levels.*[5]

How to lower lipoprotein (a):[6, 7]

Coenzyme Q-10	120-400 mg
L-carnitine	1,000-2,000 mg
Vitamin C	2,000-4,000 mg
EPA/DHA	1,000-2,000 mg
Niacin	1,000-2,000 mg
	(with the help of your physician)
L-lysine	500-1,000 mg
L-proline	500-1,000 mg
NAC	500 mg
Tocotrienols	
Estrogen replacement	
Flax seed	

Use less soy

Do not use a statin drug

11.6 C-reactive Protein

Scientists believe that infection can cause heart disease. Chlamydia, herpes, and cytomegalovirus can cause inflammation in your blood vessels and cause plaque formation. Chronic gum disease and H. pylori infection in your stomach are also causes of inflammation. C-reactive protein is an antibody-like substance that reflects the presence of a previous infection. Studies have shown that c-reactive protein can be predictive of future heart attacks even if you have a normal cholesterol level.[1, 2, 3, 4]

What causes an elevated c-reactive protein (CRP):[5, 6, 7]

- Inflammation
- Previous infection
- Obesity
- Depression
- Diabetes mellitus

How to lower c-reactive protein:[8, 9, 10, 11, 12, 13, 14, 15]

EPA/DHA	2,000-3,000 mg

Ultrainflammax (made by Metagenics, see Appendix for availability)

Vitamin E	800 IU
Coenzyme Q-10	200-300 mg

Exercise

One baby aspirin a day (ask your doctor first)

Natural cox-2 inhibitors

Grapeseed extract	100 to 200 mg
Curcumin	300 to 600 mg
Green tea	3 cups or 3 capsules

Rosemary

Quercetin	500 mg

11.7

How to stabilize plaque formation:[1]

Dietary cox-2 inhibitors previously discussed

Folic acid	2.5 mg
B12	1,000 micrograms
B6	50-100 mg
EPA/DHA	2,000 mg
Coenzyme Q-10	60 mg
Phosphatidyl choline	1,000-2,000 mg
Magnesium	600 mg
Tocotrienols	100-240 mg
Vitamin E	400-800 IU
Vitamin C	1,000-2,000 mg

12

Closed Head Injury

Supplements:[1]

EPA/DHA	3,000 mg
Flax seed	1,000 mg
Calcium citrate	1,000 mg
Vitamin E	400 IU
Zinc	25 mg twice a day
Copper	2 mg twice a day
Vitamin B6	100 mg
Vitamin B5	100 mg
Coenzyme Q-10	120 mg
Magnesium citrate	600-800 mg
Phosphatidylserine	300 mg
MVI	

Cold Symptoms

13

Supplements:

Zinc	25-50 mg
NAC	1,000-3,000
Taurine	2,000 mg
Vitamin C	2,000-5,000 mg
Echinacea	twice a day
Essential Defense	(Metagenics product see Appendix for availability)

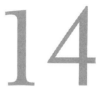

Congestive Heart Failure

Supplements:[1, 2, 3, 4, 5, 6, 7, 8, 9, 10, 11, 12, 13, 14, 15, 16]

Coenzyme Q-10	120-400 mg
L-carnitine	2,000 mg
EPA/DHA	2,000-3,000 mg
Taurine	2,000-3,000 mg
Hawthorn	160-900 mg
Magnesium	600-800 mg
Arginine	3,000-9,000
Thiamine	50-200 mg
Berberine	300-500 mg four times a day

Diabetes Mellitus 15

At The Center for Healthy Living we use a functional medicine approach to treat insulin resistance and diabetes.

- If insulin is high we decrease insulin stimulation by using a dietary approach that decreases insulin response.
- Your body's response to insulin can be made more sensitive by nutrients that modify your resonse to insulin.

We instruct our patients to use low glycemic index foods which decrease glucose response and therefore decrease insulin secretion. Low glycemic index programs also raise HDL (good) cholesterol, lower LDL (bad) cholesterol, and decrease apolipoprotein B. These benefits can be seen in as little as 4 weeks.

Insulin Resistance/ Hyperinsulinism (High Insulin)

Supplements:[1, 2, 3, 4, 5, 6, 7, 8, 9, 10, 11, 12, 13, 14, 15, 16, 17, 18, 19, 20, 21, 22, 23, 24, 25, 26, 27, 28]

EPA/DHA	2,000 mg
Vitamin E	600-800 IU
Zinc	25-50 mg
Alpha lipoic acid	200-600 mg (larger doses require physician guidance)
Taurine	1,000-3,000 mg
Chromium	400-600 micrograms

Magnesium	400- 800 mg
CLA	1,000-3,000 mg
Biotin	4-8 mg
Fiber (metafiber)	30-50 grams
Vanadium	20-50 mg
Vitamin D	400 IU
Coenzyme Q-10	30-200 mg
B complex	50 mg
Vitamin C	1,000-3,000 mg
Manganese	5-10 mg

Lentils, chickpeas, and broccoli all decrease insulin levels.

Diabetes Mellitus

Supplements:[29, 30, 31, 32, 33, 34, 35, 36, 37, 38, 39, 40, 41, 42, 43, 44, 45, 46, 47, 48]

Chromium picolinate	300-1,000 micrograms
Magnesium	400-800 mg
Vanadium	50-100 mg
Vitamin C	1,000-3,000 mg
L-carnitine	2,000-3,000 mg
Inositol	2,000-4,000 mg
Vitamin B 6	150 mg
Vitamin B12	1,000-3,000 micrograms
B complex	100 mg
EPA/DHA	2,000-3,000 mg
Gymnema sylvestre	
Fenugreek	
Alpha lipoic acid	100-300 mg (up to 1,500 mg under a doctor's care)
Carnosine	2,000 mg
GLA	240-480 mg
NAC	500-1,000 mg
Vanadium	20-50 mg
L-Taurine	1,000-1,500 mg
Zinc	20-50 mg

Copper	2-3 mg
Biotin	8-16 mg
Vitamin E	400-800 IU
Vitamin D	400 IU
Selenium	200 micrograms
Coenzyme Q-10	30-200 mg
Quercetin	300-900 mg
Ginkgo	120 mg
Bitter melon	
Fiber	Metafiber by Metagenics (see appendix)
Manganese	2-5 mg
L-arginine	1,000-5,000 mg

In our practice, for both insulin resistance and diabetes mellitus, we use a low glycemic index program and one of the following:

- Ultraglycemics is a medical food in powdered form (use as a shake) that contains many of the above nutrients. I have many of my patients combine this with Ultrameal, containing many other daily nutrient requirements. This program is also very effective for weight loss. Ultrameal and Ultraglycemics are both made by Metagenics.

- If our patients do not want to use a powder, another option is to start them on Dioxinal made by Orthomolecular. It is a capsule you take twice a day that contains chromium, alpha lipoic acid, and vanadium.

- A third approach would be for me to write them a prescription for their nutrients to lower their blood sugar, make insulin work more effectively in their body, and include all of the other daily vitamins that they would need.

Diabetic Neuropathy

Supplements:[49, 50, 51, 52, 53, 54, 55, 56, 57, 58, 59]

GLA	1,000 mg
EPA/DHA	1,000-2,000 mg
Alpha lipoic acid	300-1,500 mg under the direction of a physician
L-carnitine	2,000 mg
Vitamin B12	2,000-5,000 micrograms
Biotin	5-10 mg
Carnosine	1,000-2,000 mg
Vitamin E	400-800 IU (consult a physician if on a blood thinner)

Depression

16

It is estimated that one in five Americans has significant symptoms of depression.[1] Always see your physician and have them help with the nutritional component of treating depression. *Combining nutritional treatment and traditional medications may be countra-indicated in some cases. Do not discontinue any medication without the guidance of your doctor.* Furthermore, continual stress can counteract the beneficial affects of antidepressants and prevent a complete recovery. Consequently have your health care provider also evaluate your adrenal system.

There are nutritional deficiencies associated with depression:[2]

- Zinc
- Calcium
- Copper
- Iron
- Magnesium
- Vanadium
- Calcium
- Magnesium
- B vitamins: B12, folic acid, pyridoxine, riboflavin, thiamine, biotin

Supplements:[3, 4, 5, 6, 7, 8, 9, 10, 11, 12, 13, 14, 15, 16, 17, 18]

Magnesium	600-800 mg
Calcium	1,000 mg
Zinc	25-50 mg
EPA/DHA	1,000-3,000 mg
Vitamin A	5,000 IU
Vitamin B 12	1 mg (1,000 micrograms)
Folic acid	1, 000 micrograms
Vitamin C	1,000 mg
Phosphatidyl choline	1,000-2,000 mg
L-tyrosine	1,000-4,000 mg
Tryptophan	1,500 mg twice a day

(cannot take with anti-depressants)

St. Johns' Wort	900-1800 mg

(may cause a skin rash from sun exposure/cannot take with antidepressants, indinavir, cyclosporine, theophylline, warfarin, or ethinylestradiol)

Ginseng	500 mg
Valerian	500 mg
Alpha lipoic acid	100 mg
Coenzyme Q-10	60-100 mg
5-HTP	100 mg
Phosphatidylserine	300 mg
L-carnitine	500-3,000 mg
Inositol	1-10 grams
Centella asiatica	
Bacopa monniera	
Ashwaganda	500-1,000 mg
B complex	50-100 mg
Chromium	400 micrograms
Magnesium	400-600 mg
Copper	1-3 mg
Selenium	400 micrograms
Inositol	1,000-10,000 mg

If you have trouble with normal antidepressant doses you may need to be detoxified (see chapter on detoxification).

17

Eye Health

This chapter will cover cataract prevention and treatment, macular degeneration prevention, and the treatment of dry eyes.

Cataract Prevention and Treatment

Supplements:[1, 2, 3, 4, 5, 6, 7, 8, 9, 10, 11, 12, 13, 14, 15]

Vitamin E	400-800 IU
NAC	500 mg
Vitamin C	2,000 mg
Carnosine	1,000-2,000 mg
Alpha lipoic acid	100-300 mg
B complex vitamins	50-100 mg
Beta carotene	5,000-10,000 IU
Lutein	6 mg-12 mg
Bilberry	60 mg
Selenium	100-200 micrograms
Zinc	25-50 mg
Manganese	2 mg
Taurine	1,000 mg
Vitamin A	5,000-25,000 IU (see your doctor for doses above 10,000 IU)
Copper	1 mg
Quercetin	500-1,000 mg

Macular Degeneration

Supplements:[16, 17, 18, 19]

Vitamin A	5,000- 25,000 IU (see your doctor for doses above 10,000 IU)
Lutein	6-12 mg
Taurine	3,000 mg
Alpha lipoic acid	300-600 mg
Zinc	25-80 mg
NAC	1,000-3,000 mg
Bilberry	60 mg
Vitamin C	2,000-3,000 mg
Vitamin E	400-800 IU
B complex vitamins	100 mg
Copper	2 mg
B cartotene	10,000-25,000 IU (decrease to 8,000 IU for smokers)
L-carnitine	200 mg
EPA/DHA	1,000-2,000 mg
Coenzyme Q-10	30-60 mg
Selenium	200-300 micrograms
Ginkgo biloba	120 mg

Dry eyes

Supplements:[20]

EPA/DHA	2,000-3,000 mg

Chronic Fatigue Syndrome/ Fibromyalgia

In managing chronic fatigue syndrome it is important that you have normal intestinal health. You may need to detoxify as well. Food allergies, candida, and viral infections as well as alcohol intake may make your symptoms worse. Medications for high blood pressure, inflammation, birth control pills, antihistamines, and steroids an also make you tired.

Supplements:[1, 2, 3, 4, 5, 6, 7, 8, 9, 10, 11, 12, 13, 14, 15, 16]

EPA/DHA	1,000-3,000 mg
Coenzyme Q-10	200 mg
NAC	500-1,000 mg
Alpha lipoic acid	50-1,000 mg (above 600 mg see physician for treatment)
Selenium	100-200 micrograms
Vitamin K	100-1000 micrograms
B complex	100 mg
L-carnitine	1,000-3,000 mg
Magnesium citrate or malate	50-1,000 mg
Zinc	25-50 mg
Copper	1-3 mg

Bromelain	2,400 micrograms three to four times a day
Vitamin C	1,000-6,000 mg
Vitamin E	400-1,000 IU
Manganese	2-5 mg
GLA	240-720 mg
Curcumin	1,500-3,000 mg
L-glutamine	500-1,500 mg three times a day
Quercetin	1,500 mg
Vitamin A	5,000 IU
Malic acid	1,200-2,400 mg
MSM	3,000-15,000 mg
Probiotics	Ultra flora plus
NADH	25-10 mg
Phosphatidylserine	200-300 mg
5-HTP	100 mg
Garlic	
Ultrainflammax	(Metagenics product, see appendix)
Detoxification	

Detoxification

19

Detoxification is a process by which your body transforms toxins and medications into harmless molecules that can be eliminated. This process takes place primarily in the liver and to a smaller degree in other tissues. Science has shown that each individual has a different ability to break down toxins and detoxify medications.

Detoxification is largely accomplished in 2 phases:

- Phase I: Certain enzymes change toxins into intermediate compounds

- Phase II: Other enzymes convert the intermediate compounds created in Phase I into harmless molecules that are eliminated by your body.

Phase I is your first line of defense for the detoxification of all environmental toxins, medications, supplements (e.g., vitamins), as well as many waste products that your body produces. Decreased Phase I clearance will cause toxic accumulation in your body. Adverse reactions to medications are often due to a decreased capacity for clearing them from your system.

In Phase II detoxification large water-soluble molecules are added to toxins, usually at the reactive site formed by Phase I reactions. After Phase II modifications, the body is able to eliminate the transformed toxins in the urine or feces.

The completion of the Human Genome Project has made it possible to evaluate genetic variations that affect Phase I and

Phase II detoxification and oxidative protection. This genetically-based test is called Genovations and is available through Great Smokies Diagnostic Laboratory (see Appendix). Your doctor, through this kind of testing, can determine if your detoxification system is working.

The detoxification process is very nutrient dependent. If you are undernourished lack key vitamins or nutrients you may not be able to adequately detoxify.

Phase I detoxification requires:[1]

- Niacin
- Magnesium
- Copper
- Zinc
- Vitamin C
- Vitamins B2, B3, B6, B12
- Folic acid
- Flavonoids

Phase II detoxification requires:[2]

States of Phase II System	Required nutrients
• Glutathione conjugation	Glutathione, vitamin B6
• Amino acid conjugation	Glycine, taurine, glutamine
• Methylation	Folic acid, choline, methionine, trimethylglycine, s-adenosyl-methionine (SAMe)
• Sulfation	Cysteine, methionine, molybdenum
• Acetylation	Acetyl CoA
• Glucuronidation	Glucuronic acid

In our office we use Ultra Clear Plus (Metagenics) and milk thistle 200 mg twice a day.

Your exposure to toxins is increased by:[3]

- Eating a diet high in processed foods and fat
- Drinking tap water
- Excessive consumption of caffeine

- Excessive alcohol consumption
- Tobacco use
- Recreational drug use
- Chronic use of medications
- Lack of exercise
- Liver dysfunction
- Kidney problems
- Intestinal (gut) dysfunction
- Occupational exposure
- Using pesticides, paint, and other toxic substances without adequate protective equipment
- Living or working near areas of high vehicle traffic or industrial plants

Energy Enhancing 20

You may be tired or not have enough energy because you do not fuel your body properly. Your body's fueling system is located in the mitochondria. Your cells have up to 3,000 mitochondria each. Your mitochondrial DNA are twenty times more susceptible to damage by free radicals than the DNA located inside the nucleus of your cells. If you do not have adequate energy production, all of the functional systems of your body are impaired. Therefore, mitochondrial health is very important to maintain optimal health. *When you have symptoms of sore muscles, you have poisoned mitochondria.*

Functions of the mitochondria:[1]
- Energy production
- Synthesis of useful compounds such as steroid hormones, mRNA, mDNA
- Regulation of intracellular calcium
- Control of apoptosis (cell death)
- Removal of unwanted compounds such as urea, oxidation of lactate
- Makes glutathione
- Detoxifies cholesterol

If you have decreased omega-3-fatty acid intake you will alter what goes into the mitochondria and you produce less energy.

Energy Enhancing Nutrients

Supplements:[2]

B complex	100 mg
Alpha lipoic acid	100-300 mg
Coenzyme Q-10	100 mg
Magnesium	600 mg
Manganese	2.5-5 mg
Vitamin E	400-800 IU
Vitamin C	1,000-2,000 mg
NAC	500-1,000 mg
L-carnitine	1,000-2,000 mg
Zinc	25 mg
NADH	5-10 mg

21

Gall Bladder Symptoms

Supplements:[1]

Taurine	500 mg twice a day

Bitters
Taraxacum (dandelion root)
Chelidonium (greater celandine)
Cynara (artichoke leaf)
Rosemarinus (rosemary)
Mentha (peppermint)
Humulus (hops)

22

Gut Repair

The health of your intestinal tract is very important.

Your gut is four things:
- It is a bioreactor taking in foods and breaking them down.
- It is the information center of the body because it is a signaling organism.
- It is an immune organ since *more than 50 percent of your immune system is located in your gut.*
- It is a brain with two-thirds of your serotonin being produced in your gut.

What causes you to have poor gut health?[1]
- Infections: viral, bacterial, protozoa, parasites, fungi
- Alcohol
- Tobacco
- Medications: non-steroidal anti-inflammatory drugs such as ibuprofen, antibiotics
- Antacids
- Excess sugar intake
- Poor nutrition
- Stress
- Free radical production
- Low acid
- Decrease in digestive enzymes
- Low bile production

- Food allergies
- Travel
- Diabetes
- Altitude

These agents create dysbiosis, a state of gut dysfunction.

Dysbiosis causes:
- Loss of good bacteria
- Loss of vitamin production
- Loss of detoxification
- Overgrowth of "bad bacteria" and yeast
- Malabsorption
- Leaky gut syndrome

Malabsorption is a condition where vitamins, minerals, fatty acids, amino acids, and other nutrients are not taken across the intestinal wall into your blood stream. Your body can also develop increased intestinal permeability where substances including medications and toxins that should not be crossing into your blood stream are allowed to do so. This is called leaky gut syndrome.

These nutrients help repair your gut:[2, 3, 4]

L-glutamine	2,000 mg-10,000 mg
EPA/DHA	500 mg-1,000 mg three times a day
Quercitin	500 mg three times a day
Zinc	10-20 mg three times a day
GLA	500 mg three times a day
Pantothenic acid	100-200 mg three times a day
Vitamin A	5,000 to 25,000 IU (only up to 8,000 IU if smoker)
Probiotics	Ultra flora plus
NAC	500 mg
MSM	1,000 mg three times a day or Ultra-inflammax (Metagenics product see Appendix for availability)

Vitamin E	400 IU
Fiber	Metafiber (see appendix under Metagenics)
Vitamin C	1,000 mg

Pancreatic enzymes

Our patients with poor gut health go through a program called the 4R program:[5]

- Remove: allergens, antigens, pathogens, parasites
- Reinoculate: with good bacteria: pre and probiotics
- Replace: with symbiotic flora: pre and probiotics
- Repair: gut mucosal nutrients

We use Ultra Clear Plus and Ultra Clear Sustain and other products by Metagenics for this purpose. For a health professional who can help you through the Four R Program see the Introduction.

Your health care provider can order a comprehensive digestive stool analysis (CDSA) from Great Smokies Laboratory to identify areas of gut repair that need treatment.

Avoid non-steroidal anti-inflammatory drugs such as aspirin and ibuprofen. Likewise avoid antibiotics as much as possible since all of these will cause increased intestinal permeability and a reoccurrence of leaky gut syndrome.

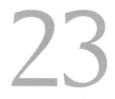

Hair Thinning

Supplements:

- Saw palmetto
- Nettles
- Indole-3-carbinol
- Rosemary

24

Migraine Headaches —Prevention

Supplements:[1, 2, 3, 4, 5, 6, 7, 8, 9, 10, 11]

Riboflavin	200-400 mg
Feverfew	100 mg
Magnesium	600-800 mg
EPA/DHA	1,000-2,000 mg
B complex	100 mg
Coenzyme Q-10	60-150 mg
L-Carnitine	1,000-3,000 mg
Vitamin C	1,000-3,000 mg
Calcium	500-1,000 mg
Selenium	200 micrograms
Vitamin E	400-800 IU
Vitamin D	400 IU
Zinc	25 mg
Curcumin	100-1,000 mg
Probiotics	Ultra flora plus

25

Hepatitis C

Supplements:[1, 2, 3, 4, 5]

Alpha lipoic acid	300-600 mg
Phosphatidyl choline	2,000-10,000 mg
Probiotics	Ultra flora plus
NAC	1,000 mg
Vitamin C	1,000-5,000 mg
Vitamin E	400 IU
Lysine	1,000-3,000 mg
B complex	50 mg
Folic acid	1,000 micrograms
Vitamin B12	1,000-2,000 micrograms
Selenium	200-400 micrograms
Coenzyme Q-10	100-400 mg
Carnitine	500-3,000 mg
Taurine	1,000-3,000 mg
Olive leaf extract	1-3 capsules
Silymarin	100-300 mg
Astragalus	1-3 ml of tincture or capsule extract

Avoid high doses of vitamin A or beta carotene. Also avoid niacin supplementation greater than 100 mg.

26

High Blood Pressure (Hypertension)

One out of every four adults in the U.S. has high blood pressure.[1] If your blood pressure remains elevated you are more likely to have a stroke, heart disease, or congestive heart failure than someone who has a normal blood pressure.

Risk factors for high blood pressure:[2]
- Age (50 percent of adults over the age of 60)
- Genetics
- Race (more common in Blacks)
- Alcohol abuse
- Drug use
    Amphetamine-like medications
    Cocaine
    Steroids
    Cyclosporine
    Decongestants
    Ephedra
    Erythropoietin
    MAO inhibitors and phenothiazines (antidepressants and
      medications for psychosis)
    Non-steroidal anti-inflammatory drugs such as aspirin and
      ibuprofen
    COX- inhibitors (for arthritis)
    Birth control pills

- Poor diet
    - High sodium
    - Saturated fat
    - Trans fatty acids
    - Sugar
    - Refined carbohydrates
    - Caffeine
- Lack of exercise
- Obesity
- Smoking
- Stress
- Education and income (more education and higher income the lower the blood pressure)
- Free radical production

Medications treat the symptoms of high blood pressure, but they do not treat the cause of the problem. Getting at the root of the situation requires nutrition, change in eating habits, and life style changes. For a more in depth look at this subject, read *Hypertension and Nutrition* by Eric Braverman, M.D. Dr. Braverman points out the following sad facts concerning blood pressure medications:[3]

- Fifty percent of all elderly patients on Thiazide diuretics show severe potassium or magnesium deficiencies.
- Diuretics can increase the possibility of severe life-threatening arrhythmias and raise cholesterol, triglycerides, and other dangerous fat factors in the blood. Patients on diuretics have an increased risk of death due to heart attack or sudden death and diuretics can damage the kidneys.
- Beta blockers worsen asthma and increase depression (25 percent of all patients on blockers eventually must be treated with antidepressant medications).
- Alpha-blockers are not particularly helpful in long-term treatment of high blood pressure. They can cause sedation, constipation, and dizziness.

- Hydralazine decreases your body's stores of manganese and can lead to seizures.
- Most medications for high blood pressure interfere with normal brain function, decrease alertness and memory, and can cause premature senility symptoms if you are over 60. These side effects are greatly reduced by nutritional supplementation.
- Angiotensin-2 inhibitors may decrease your body stores of trace minerals that protect your immune system such as copper, zinc, and selenium.
- Angiotensin-2 blockers worsen the quality of life for 30-40 percent of all patients.

What else can you do?

You can begin by working with a doctor to help replace your blood pressure medications with supplements that work like drugs but do not have side effects. *I do not recommend that you stop taking your blood pressure medication without working with a physician trained in functional medicine that can help you change your life style to decrease your risk of heart disease and blood pressure.* Stress, poor food choices, smoking, excess salt, sugar, and alcohol, along with caffeine can be some of the contributing factors. Exercise is also very important to lower blood pressure.

The following are some of the supplements that have been effectively used to treat hypertension. There are many natural nutrients that can substitute or be used to augment antihypertensive medications so that lower dosages can be used. See a health care provider for assistance in this area.

Supplements:[4]

Diuretics

- Hawthorn berry
- Vitamin B 6
- Taurine
- Celery
- GLA
- Vitamin C
- Potassium
- Magnesium
- Calcium
- Protein
- Fiber
- Coenzyme Q-10
- L-carnitine

Direct vasodilators

- Omega-3-fatty acids
- MUFA (omega-9 fatty acids)
- Potassium
- Magnesium
- Calcium
- Soy
- Fiber
- Garlic
- Flavonoids
- Vitamin C
- Vitamin E
- Coenzyme Q-10
- L-arginine
- Taurine
- Celery
- Alpha lipoic acid

Angiotensin Converting Enzyme Inhibitors (ACE 1):

- Garlic
- Seaweed
- Tuna
- Sardine
- Hawthorn berry
- Pycnogenol
- Casein
- Hydrolyzed whey protein
- Gelatin
- Sake
- Omega-3-fatty acids
- Egg yolks
- Zinc
- Hydrolyzed wheat germ isolate

Beta Blockers

- Hawthorn berry

Central Alpha Agonist

- Taurine
- Potassium
- Zinc
- Sodium restriction
- Protein
- Fiber
- Vitamin C
- Vitamin B6
- Coenzyme Q-10
- Celery
- GLA/DHA
- Garlic

Calcium Channel Blockers

- Alpha lipoic acid
- Vitamin C
- Vitamin B6
- Magnesium
- NAC
- Vitamin E
- Hawthorn berry
- Celery
- Omega-3-fatty acids
- Calcium
- Garlic

Angiotensin Receptor Blockers

- Potassium
- Fiber
- Garlic
- Vitamin C
- Vitamin B6
- Coenzyme Q-10
- Celery
- GLA and DGLA

Supplements to lower blood pressure:[5, 6, 7, 8, 9, 10, 11, 12, 13, 14, 15, 16]

Calcium	1,000-1,200 mg
Magnesium	600-800 mg
Vitamin D	400-800 IU
EPA/DHA	3,000-4,000 mg
Vitamin C	1,000 mg
Coenzyme Q-10	60-120 mg
B complex	100 mg
Zinc	25 mg
L-arginine	5,000 mg
Hawthorn berry	160-900 mg
L-taurine	1,000-1,500 mg
L-carnitine	1,000-2,000 mg
NAC	1,000 mg
Alpha lipoic acid	100-200 mg
Lycopene	10 mg
Vitamin E	400-800 IU
Celery seed powder	500 mg
Garlic	10,000 micrograms

Diet is also important. A low salt program with low glycemic index carbohydrates, high fiber, and an abundance of flavonoids has been shown to be helpful. Lentils, hazelnuts, walnuts, and peanuts contain arginine which will also lower your blood pressure.[17, 18, 19, 20]

Two other books I highly recommend are: *What Your Doctor May Not Tell You About Hypertension* by Mark Houston, M.D. and *Lower Your Blood Pressure In Eight Weeks* by Stephen Sinatra, M.D.[21, 22]

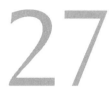

Bowel Disease

IBS (Irritable Bowel Syndrome)
Crohn's Disease
Ulcerative Colitis

Irritable bowel syndrome affects 30 million people in the United States.[1]

The following are signs and symptoms of IBS:
- Constipation and or diarrhea
- Cramps
- Gas
- Urgency
- Nausea

Causes of irritable bowel syndrome:[2]
- Diet (wheat, corn, dairy, coffee, tea, citrus: cause the most symptoms)
- Sugar
- Stress
- Bacterial overgrowth (due to excessive use of antibiotics)
- Yeast overgrowth
- Lactose intolerance
- Parasites

Supplements:[3, 4, 5, 6, 7, 8, 9, 10]

Fiber
Water
Decrease simple sugars
4 R program
Ultrainflammax by Metagenics (see Appendix)
Inflamablox by Orthomolecular (see Appendix)

Probiotics	Ultra flora plus
Glutamine	1,000-40,000 mg
Vitamin A	5,000-10,000 IU
Folic acid	800 micrograms
Vitamin B12	800 micrograms
Zinc	25-75 mg
Vitamin C	1,000-3,000 mg
Vitamin E	200-400 IU
Magnesium	400-800 mg

DGL (deglycyrrhizinated licorice) 1-4 tablets
 (do not take with high blood pressure)

EPA/DHA	1,000-2,000 mg
GLA	240-720 mg
Boswella extract	2-3 capsules
Pancreatic enzymes	1-2 capsules one hour after eating
Peppermint oil	
Colostrum	
Quercetin	500-2,000 mg
Garlic	900 mg
Olive leaf	1,000 mg

Avoid sugar and grain. Do not eat crackers, cakes, cookies, bread, pasta, flour, cereals, rolls, potatoes, yams, parsnips, chickpeas, and soybeans.

Immune Building 28

The following things can affect your immune system:[1]
- Lack of sleep
- Toxin exposure
- Age
- Infection
- Stress
- Nutrition depletion
- Overuse of antibiotics

Supplements:[2, 3, 4, 5, 6, 7, 8, 9, 10, 11, 12]

Zinc	15-50 mg
Vitamin A	5,000-25,000 IU

(not when pregnant and not for more than 3 months at more than 10,000 IU, smokers do not use more than 10,000 IU at any time)

Selenium	400 micrograms
Probiotics	Ultra flora plus
Taurine	1,000-3,000 mg
Vitamin C	1,000-20,000 mg
Vitamin E	400-800 IU
Carnitine	1,000-3,000 mg
Coenzyme Q-10	50-300 mg
Mixed carotenoids	5,000-50,000 IU (more than 10,000 IU requires doctors care)

B complex	50 mg
NAC	500-2,000 mg
Glutamine	1,000-10,000 mg
Magnesium	400-600 mg
GLA	240-480 mg
Curcuminoids	1,000-1,500 mg
Chlorella/spirulina	1-2 tablespoons
Echinacea	2 tablets (short term use only)
Astragalus	1,000-2,000 mg or 1-4 droppers full of tincture
Colostrum	
Garlic	300-900 mg
Transfer factor	
Green tea extract	1,000 mg

In our office we use Essential Defense made by Metagenics (see Appendix for availability).

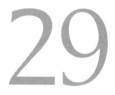

Insomnia

Insomnia is the perception or complaint of inadequate or poor quality sleep, which may result in daytime tiredness, lack of energy, difficulty concentrating, and/or irritability.[1] One-half of all Americans have experienced insomnia.[2] Drowsiness due to lack of a good nights sleep interferes with the daily activities of 37 percent of all adults.[3]

Factors that contribute to insomnia:[4, 5, 6]

- Diet
    Caffeinated beverages
    Food allergies
    Food additives
- Illness
    Urinary disorders
    Nasal and sinus problems
    Hiatal hernia/reflux esophagitis
    Anxiety disorder
    Depression
    Asthma
    Gallbladder disease
    Chronic pain

- Hormonal
    Thyroid dysfunction
    Growth hormone loss
    Progesterone loss
    Testosterone loss (men)
    Estrogen loss (women)
    Elevated cortisol
- Medication
    Asthma medications
    Sleeping pills
    Blood pressure medications
    Synthetic progestins
- Exercise (lack of)
- Sleep apnea
- Light
- Shift work
- Nutritional deficiency
    Niacin deficiency
    Magnesium deficiency
    Copper deficiency or excess
    Low iron
    Tryptophan deficiency
    Vitamin B6 deficiency
- Chemical exposure (over 100 chemicals that can decrease sleep)

Supplements:[7, 8, 9, 10, 11, 12, 13]

Magnesium	600 mg
GABA plus	300-900 mg
5-HTP	100-200 mg
Inositol	1,000 mg
Melatonin	1-6 mg

Lemon balm (cannot use if pregnant or have glaucoma)

Passion flower (cannot take if on MAO inhibitor or pregnant)
Jujube (cannot take if pregnant)
Astragalus (cannot take if gum allergy)
Chamomile (may have allergy to if allergic to ragweed)

In our office we use Serenagen by Metagenics and Natural ZZZ by Orthomolecular (for availability see Appendix).

30

Leg Cramps

Supplements:[1]

Vitamin E	400-800 IU
Calcium	1,000 mg
Magnesium	600-800 mg
Potassium	As prescribed by your doctor
Niacin	100 mg
EPA/DHA	1,000 mg

Liver Health

31

Functions of your liver:

- Maintains red blood cells
- Removes bacteria from your body
- Stores blood
- Produces proteins responsible for maintaining your blood pressure
- Synthesizes clotting factors
- Helps metabolize foods
- Detoxifies poisons and medications
- Stores vitamins and minerals
- Produces bile

Supplements:[1, 2, 3, 4, 5, 6]

Milk thistle	100-300 mg
Dandelion	100 mg
Zinc	25 mg
Magnesium	400-600 mg
Vitamin E	400 IU
B complex	50 mg
Coenzyme Q-10	100-400 mg
Alpha lipoic acid	100-600 mg
Artichoke	
Hesperidin	
Phosphatidyl choline	1,000-3,000 mg

Quercetin	500 mg
L-carnitine	500-3,000 mg
Isothiocyanates (cruciferous vegetables)	
NAC	1,000 mg
Carosol (rosemary)	
Limonene (lemon oil)	
Perillyl alcohol (cherries)	
Curcuminoids (tumeric)	
L-taurine	1,000-3,000 mg
Selenium	200-400 micrograms
Vitamin B12	1,000-2,000 micrograms
Folic acid	1,000 micrograms
Inositol	1,000 mg
Vitamin C	1,000-5,000 mg

32

Memory-Enhancing Brain Nutrient Program

Factors that affect your memory:[1, 2, 3, 4]

- Nutrition
- Free radical production (oxidative stress)
  - Alcohol
  - Bacterial waste
  - Smoking
  - Stress
  - Food allergies
  - Diabetes
  - White blood cell activity
  - MSG
  - Trauma or injury
  - Medications
  - Viruses
  - Lead, mercury, cadmium
  - Excess iron, manganese, copper
  - Toxic chemicals (benzene, toluene, etc.)
  - Liver disease
  - Intestinal dysbiosis (imbalance of gut organisms)
  - Normal oxygen using capacity

- Mental and physical stress (elevated or decreased cortisol levels)
- Medications
  - Analgesics (pain medications)
  - Antiarrhythmic drugs
  - Antibiotics
  - Anticonvulsants
  - Antidepressants
  - Antihistamines and decongestants
  - Antihypertensive drugs
  - Levodopa
  - Steroids
  - Muscle relaxants
  - Sedatives
  - Statin medications
- Recreational drugs
- Education and other environmental stimuli
- Genetics

The following suggested protocols were developed by Dr. Robert Goldman, founder and president of the National Academy of Sports Medicine, and cofounder of the American Academy of Anti-Aging Medicine. I personally follow this program and have found it very useful in my patients. For more information on this subject, read *Brain Fitness* by Robert Goldman, M.D., D.O.[5] Other references for the programs below include:[6, 7, 8, 9, 10, 11]

Memory-enhancing Brain Nutrient Program:

Choline	50-100 mg
Folic acid	500-800 micrograms
Ginkgo biloba	50-150 mg
(cannot take ginkgo if you take a blood thinner)	
Magnesium	600-800 mg
Phosphatidyl choline	200-500 mg
Phosphatidylserine	300-500 mg

B complex vitamins	100 mg
Vitamin C	1,000-2,000 mg
Zinc	30-50 mg
Alpha lipoic acid	100 mg
EPA/DHA	1,000 mg
Coenzyme Q-10	60 mg

Mental Alertness Brain Nutrient Program:

Glutamine	1,000-2,000 mg
Tyrosine	1,000-2,000 mg
Acetyl-L-carnitine	50-100 mg
Ginseng	200-500 mg
Ginkgo biloba	50-100 mg
(cannot take if you are on a blood thinner)	
Pantothenic acid	50-100 mg
Phosphatidyl choline	1,000-4,000 mg
Magnesium	600 mg
Phosphatidylserine	300-500 mg
Vitamin C	3,000 mg
Zinc	30 mg
B complex	50-100 mg
EPA/DHA	1,000 mg
Coenzyme Q-10	60 mg

Alzheimer's Protection Brain Nutrient Program:

Acetyl-L-carnitine	1,000-2,000 mg
Vitamin A	5,000 IU
Mixed carotinoid	5,000 IU
Vitamin C	1,000-2,000 mg
Vitamin E	400-800 IU
(may need to lower dose of on a blood thinner)	
NAC	1,000 mg
Selenium	100-200 micrograms
B complex vitamins	100 mg
Phosphatidyl choline	1,000-4,000 mg

Coenzyme Q-10	100-200 mg
Ginkgo biloba	100-250 mg

(cannot take if on a blood thinner)

Alpha lipoic acid	100-200 mg
Phosphatidylserine	200-300 mg
EPA/DHA	1,000-2,000 mg
Vitamin B12	1,000 micrograms
Folic acid	800 micrograms
Vinpocetine	5 mg three times a day
Resveratrol	20 mg

Multiple Sclerosis (MS)

33

Diet does affect MS greatly. A low fat program with no red meat and no dairy has been shown in several studies to decrease the number of new MS lesions.[1, 2, 3, 4, 5, 6, 7, 8] Adding "good" fats such as omega 3 fatty acids does improve or stabilize the condition. Abstension from alcohol has also been proven to be helpful. I do recommend that you have your doctor measure your essential fatty acids through Great Smokies Diagnostic Laboratory. An excellent book on this subject is *Brain Recovery.Com* by David Perlmutter, M.D.[9]

Supplements:[10, 11, 12, 13, 14, 15]

B12	1,000 micrograms
EPA/DHA	1,000-3,000 mg
GLA	300 mg
Vitamin B3	50 mg
Vitamin B6	50 mg
Vitamin C	1,000 mg
Vitamin E	400 IU
Vitamin D	400-800 IU
Ginkgo biloba	30 mg
(cannot take if on a blood thinner)	
Alpha lipoic acid	100-300 mg
NAC	200 mg

Coenzyme Q-10	30-100 mg
NADH	10 mg
Phosphatidylserine	100-200 mg
Magnesium	400 mg
Zinc	10 mg
Folic acid	500 micrograms
Selenium	200 micrograms
L-Carnitine	500-3,000 mg
Copper	1-2 mg

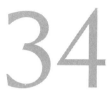

Muscle Development

In order to have muscle development you need four basic materials:

- Glucose
- Fat
- Amino acids
- Normal hormone levels

Amino acids are needed to make the proteins that form your muscles. Insulin that is not working effectively in your body slows muscle development and promotes fat formation. (See insulin resistance). Have your physician measure your amino acid levels if you want to optimize your muscle development. (Great Smokies Diagnostic Laboratory, see Appendix).

Supplements:

Chromium	600-1,200 micrograms

Sore Muscles After Exercise

Supplements:

Zinc	25-50 mg
Carnitine	1,000-2,000 mg
Coenzyme Q-10	60-100 mg
MSM	1,000 mg three times a day

35

Osteoporosis

At least 1.2 million fractures occur in the U.S. each year due to osteoporosis.[1] It is not just a woman's disease. One-third of the cases of osteoporosis in the U.S. occur in men.

Things that increase your risk of osteoporosis:[2, 3, 4, 5, 6, 7, 8]

- If you intake excess protein (more than 100 mg a day) you increase your risk of osteoporosis. When protein is broken down, very acidic products are formed that accumulate in the urine. When this occurs calcium is mobilized and taken from your bone.

- If you take antacids on a daily basis, or drink soft drinks regularly you also increase your risk of bone loss.

- Caffeine increases calcium loss. If you drink three cups of coffee a day you cause a 45 mg calcium loss. Coffee contains twenty-nine different acids which also draw calcium out from your bones. Be aware that many medications both prescription and non-prescription contain caffeine. More than 1,000 over-the-counter medications contain caffeine including weight loss products, cold preparations, pain relievers, and allergy products.

- Foods that contain oxalic acid such as spinach, chard, beet, dandelion greens, rhubarb, asparagus, and chocolate bind with calcium and decrease its absorption.

- Grains contain phytic acid which combines with calcium to lower its absorption.

- Insoluble fiber also interferes with calcium absorption.
- If your homocysteine level is high it can interfere with proper bone formation. Have your doctor measure your homocysteine level.
- Excessive vitamin A intake and thyroid medication that is excess can both lead to osteoporosis.
- Sugar
- Excess alcohol intake
- Immobility (lack of weight bearing exercise)
- Smoking
- Genetics
- Medications
  Steroids
  Seizure medications
  Anticoagulants (blood thinners)
  Some cancer chemotherapy medications
  Lithium
  Tetracycline
  Loop diuretics

Supplements:[9, 10, 11, 12, 13, 14, 15, 16, 17, 18, 19, 20, 21, 22]

Vitamin D	400-800 IU
Calcium	500-1,200 mg
Magnesium	400-800 mg
Manganese	5-10 mg
Potassium	through diet
Ipriflavone	100-300 mg (300-600 mg in osteoporosis)
Zinc	25 mg
Copper	1-2 mg
Vitamin K	150 micrograms
Vitamin C	1,000 mg
Boron	5-10 mg
Folic acid	500 micrograms

Vitamin B12	100 micrograms
EPA/DHA	500-1,000 mg
GLA	240 mg

Calcium hydroxyapatite has been shown in clinical trials to enhance bone formation. Calcium citrate is also a good form of calcium to use. Calcium carbonate is much less absorbed. *With calcium it is very important to use a pharmaceutical grade product. Many of the calcium products sold inside the U.S. contain contaminants such as lead and mercury.*

Parkinson's Disease

36

Parkinson's Disease is associated with a defect in the function of your mitochondria, the energy producing parts of your cells. Dr. David Perlmutter in his book *Brain Recovery.com* has an excellent discussion of various treatments of Parkinson's Disease.[1] Liver toxicity is associated with Parkinson's Disease. Have your physician run a hepatic detoxification profile available by Great Smokies Laboratory to see if this is a problem.

Supplements:[2, 3, 4, 5, 6, 7, 8]

Coenzyme Q-10	120 mg
NADH	5-10 mg
Phosphatidylserine	300-500 mg
Vitamin E	800-1,200 IU
(if you are taking a blood thinner you may not be able to take high doses of vitamin E)	
Vitamin C	1,000-5,000 mg
Alpha lipoic acid	100-600 mg
Vitamin D	400 IU
NAC	500-2,000 mg
Acetyl-L-Carnitine	1,500-3,000 mg
Gingko biloba	240-360 mg
(cannot take if on a blood thinner)	
Silymarin	100-300 mg
Probiotics	Ultra flora plus
Selenium	200-400 micrograms
Grape seed extract	50-400 mg
Bilberry	100-300 mg

Periodontal Disease 37

Supplements:[1, 2]

Coenzyme Q-10 brushed on gums
Coenzyme Q-10 taken by mouth   120 mg
Carnitine   1,000-2,000 mg
Vitamin A   25,000 IU
(this dose should be used short term. If you smoke use 10,000
IU. If you have liver disease contact your doctor before begin-
ning)
Probiotics   Ultra flora plus
Coenzyme Q-10   (under age 30)   50-100 mg
                            (over age 30)   100-200 mg
Vitamin C   2,000-5,000 mg
Vitamin E   400 IU
Zinc   25 mg
Copper   2 mg
Vitamin B6   100 mg

Men's Health

Herbs to help the prostate:[1]

- Bachu
- Cernilton
- Couch grass
- Cram bark
- Cranberry
- Dong quai (cannot be used if you have diabetes)
- Echinacea (short term use for prostatitis)
- Garlic
- Goldenseal (do not use if you have high or low blood pressure, heart disease, diabetes, glaucoma, stoke)
- Juniper
- Marshmallow
- Pipsissew
- Rosemary
- Skullcap
- Siberian ginseng
- Valerian
- Pycnogenol
- Saw palmetto
- Pygeum africanum
- Urtica dioica/stinging nettles

BPH (Benign Prostatic Hypertrophy/ Enlarged Prostate):[2, 3, 4, 5, 6, 7, 8, 9, 10]

Soy

Zinc	35-50 mg
Copper	1-2 mg
Saw palmetto	320 mg
GLA	500 mg
Selenium	100-200 micrograms
Vitamin E	400-800 IU

(may need a lower dose if on a blood thinner)

Vitamin A	5,000-10,000 IU
Vitamin C	1,000 mg
Vitamin B complex	50-100 mg

Glycine, alanine, glutamic acid are amino acids that help with an enlarged prostate

Flax seed	1,000 mg
Lycopene	10 mg
Soy Isoflavones	50-300 mg

Urtica dioica (stinging nettles)

Yes, men you produce estrogen also. Men need a small amount of estrogen since it is beneficial to the male brain. Men make estrogen from testosterone with the help of an enzyme called aromatase. Too much estrogen in males is associated with heart disease since it causes increases in clotting factors as well as narrowing of the coronary arteries in men. Too much estrogen in males will also have a neutering effect on men.[11]

Causes of estrogen elevation in men:[12]

- Increase in aromatase activity
- Alteration in liver function
- Zinc deficiency
- Obesity
- Overuse of alcohol

- Drug-induced estrogen imbalance

    Pain/anti-inflammatory drugs: ibuprofen, acetaminophen, aspirin, propoxeyphene

    Antibiotics: sulfas, tetracyclines, penicillins, cefazolins, erythromycins, floxcins, isoniazid

    Antifungal drugs: miconazole, itraconazole, fluconazole, ketoconazole

    Cholesterol lowering drugs: statins

    Antidepressants: fluoxitine, fluvoxamine, paroxetine, sertraline

    Antipsychotic medicines: thorazine, haloperidol

    Heart and blood pressure medicine: propranolol, quinidine, amiodarone, coumadin, methyldopa, calcium channel blockers

    Antacids: omeprazole, cimetidine

    Vitamins and nutrients: high-dose vitamin E, general dietary deficiencies and malnutrition, grapefruit

    Abusive substances: alcohol, amphetamines, marijuana, cocaine
- Ingestions of estrogen enhancing food or environmental substances

Things that decrease estrogen levels in men:[13, 14]
- High-dose vitamin C
- Vitamin K
- Niacin
- Soy products
- Vegetarian diets
- Cruciferous vegetables (broccoli, cauliflower, kale, Brussels sprouts)
- Shellfish (oysters)
- Resveratrol (grape skin compound)

39

Skin Disorders

Psoriasis/Eczema/Acne

Supplements:[1, 2, 3, 4]

EPA/DHA	1,000-3,000 mg
Evening primrose oil	500-1,000 mg
Glucosamine	1,000 mg
Vitamin D	400-800 IU
Milk thistle	200 mg
Dandelion	100 mg
L-taurine	2,000 mg
Zinc	25-75 mg
Copper	2-3 mg
Probiotics	Ultra flora plus
Vitamin A	50,000-300,000 IU
(under physician supervision only)	
B complex	50-100 mg
Vitamin C	1,000-3,000 mg
Vitamin E	400 IU
MSM	3,000-10,000 mg
Tea tree oil	apply directly to blemishes once or twice a day

Smoking

40

Smoking puts severe oxidative stress on your body. Nitrous oxide in cigarette smoke depletes your body of vitamins C and E. Therefore it takes 2 to 3 times the amount of vitamin C to get the same blood levels as nonsmokers.[1] Cadmium may be sprayed on tobacco to get rid of fungus. Cadmium decreases selenium availability to your body and decreases zinc metabolism.

Supplements:[2, 3]

Vitamin C	3,000-5,000 mg
L-carnitine	1,000 mg
Vitamin E	400-800 IU
(may need a lower dose if on a blood thinner)	
Selenium	100 micrograms
Coenzyme Q-10	90 mg
Alpha lipoic acid	100 mg
NAC	1,000 mg

41

Sports Nutrition

Endurance Training

Supplements:[1, 2, 3, 4, 5, 6, 7, 8, 9, 10, 11, 12, 13, 14, 15, 16, 17, 18, 19, 20, 21, 22, 23, 24, 25, 26, 27]

NAC	1,000-2,000 mg
Vitamin A	5,000 IU
Beta carotene	5,000 IU
Vitamin C	2,000-10,000 mg
Vitamin E	400-800 IU
Calcium	800-1,200 mg
Zinc	10-60 mg
Selenium	200 micrograms
Coenzyme Q-10	100-200 mg
L-carnitine	3,000-10,000 mg
DMG	125-250 mg
Phosphatidylserine	100-300 mg
Magnesium	400-600 mg
MVI	
Alpha lipoic acid	100-200 mg (600 mg if marathon race)
Flax seed oil	1 tablespoon
Ginkgo biloba	40-60 mg
(cannot take if on a blood thinner)	
EPA/DHA	1,000-2,000 mg
Chromium	200-1,200 micrograms

Siberian ginseng	1,000 mg
Reishi mushroom	1,000 mg
L-taurine	1,000 mg
L-glutamine	1,000-3,000 mg
L-glycine	1,000 mg

Strength Training

Supplements (references same as above):

Zinc	25 mg
Magnesium	400-600 mg
Arginine	2,000-10,000 mg
Glutamine	4,000-10,000 mg
Vitamin C	1,000 mg
Vitamin E	400 IU
Chromium	400-1,200 micrograms
L-taurine	1,000 mg
NAC	500-1,000 mg
L-carnitine	3,000-10,000 mg

Always make sure that you do not over train.

Signs of overtraining:[28]

- Slow recovery
- Poor performance, feeling trapped in a routine
- Loss of purpose, energy, and competitive drive
- Fatigue during exercise and rest
- Insomnia, loss of appetite, excessive sweating
- Increased susceptibility to infections
- Anxiety, irritability, emotional liability
- Loss of libido
- Muscle pain

Stress Reduction/ Adrenal Burnout

42

When you are stressed, your adrenal hormones, DHEA and cortisol change. At first, both cortisol and DHEA increase with stress and at that time you have no symptoms. Later on, cortisol increases and DHEA decreases. At this point you feel stressed, anxious, and have mood swings. Finally, if you stay stressed for an extended period of time, your adrenal hormones can no longer be made and you develop adrenal burnout. At this point, you feel depressed and exhausted. Prayer, meditation, yoga, qigong, relaxation therapies, adequate sleep, regular exercise, and a program to decrease sugar and caffeine intake are all important.

Symptoms of adrenal burnout: [1]
- Fatigue (worse in evenings and with stress)
- Restlessness
- Irritability
- Absent-minded
- Dizziness
- Hypoglycemia
- Salt cravings
- Crave sugar
- Crave spices
- Tachycardia (fast heart rate)/palpitations
- Pale, cold, clammy skin

- Inability to concentrate
- Frustration
- Insomnia
- Allergies
- Nervousness
- Depression
- Weakness
- Lightheadedness
- Headaches

Causes of adrenal stress:[2]

- Physical trauma
- Poor diet
- Lack of sleep
- Pregnancy
- Emotional trauma
- Depression
- Infections
- Anxiety
- Prescription drugs
- Chemical toxins
- Excess exercise

Adrenal Support

Supplements:[3, 4, 5, 6, 7, 8, 9, 10, 11, 12, 13] (for all protocols below)

Soy	
Glycyrrhiza	600 mg twice a day
Ashwaghanda	160 mg twice a day
Rheumania root	2,000 mg twice a day
Ginseng	200 mg twice a day
Cordyceps	400 mg twice a day
Rhodiola	50 mg twice a day
Vitamin B6	100 mg twice a day
Vitamin C	1,000-2,000 mg
DHEA	(as prescribed by your doctor)
Carnitine	1,000-3,000 mg

If You Are Stressed and Wired, Anxious

Supplements:

Holy basil	
Ashwagandha	1,000 mg
Bacopa	
Rheumania root	2,000 mg twice a day
B vitamins	100 mg
GABA	300-1,200 mg
EPA/DHA	2,000 mg
Magnesium	400-600 mg
Taurine	2,000 mg
Chromium	300 micrograms
Inositol	50-100 mg

If You Are Stressed and Fatigued

Supplements:

Ginseng	200 mg twice a day
Cordyceps	400 mg twice a day
Rhodiola	50 mg twice a day
B vitamins	100 mg
Holy basil	
Ashwagandha	1,000 mg
Bacopa	

At our office we use Adreset and Serenagen, both made by Metagenics, which have many of the nutrients listed above in them (see Appendix).

Stroke Recovery 43

These nutrients can be used immediately after stroke and are also effective months and years later.

Supplements:[1, 2]

Coenzyme Q-10	150-200 mg
Phosphatidylserine	100 mg
NADH	10 mg
Acetyl-L-carnitine	400 mg
Vinpocetine	10 mg
Folic acid	800 micrograms
Vitamin B3	100 mg
Vitamin B6	100 mg
Vitamin B12	200 micrograms
GPC (Glycerophosphocholine)	300-1,200 mg

Sun Exposure

44

It only takes a brief period of time in the sun in order for your body to become depleted of antioxidants. After only 10 minutes, there is a 50 percent reduction in the concentration of vitamin E in your skin. Therefore, if you are going to be out in the sun any length of time the following nutrients would be helpful.

Supplements:[1]

Vitamin E	400 IU
Coenzyme Q-10	30-60 mg
Vitamin C	1,000 mg
NAC	500 mg

Surgery: Pre and Post Operative

45

Supplements:[1, 2, 3, 4, 5]

Zinc	25-50 mg
Vitamin A	25, 000 IU
Vitamin C	1,000-2,000 mg
L-carnitine	1,500 mg
Phosphatidylserine	300 mg
Grape seed extract	200 mg
Probiotics	Ultra flora plus
Coenzyme Q-10	30 mg
L-glutamine	3,000-5,000 mg
Alpha lipoic acid	200-300 mg
Arginine	1,000-5,000 mg
MSM	3,000-10,000 mg
Magnesium	400 mg
Selenium	200 micrograms
NAC	1,000 mg
Taurine	1,000-3,000 mg
Gota Kola	1-3 capsules

Supplements to avoid 2 weeks before and after surgery:[6]

- Vitamin E
- Garlic
- Cayenne
- Ginkgo
- St. John's wort
- EPA/DHA

Thyroid Disease 46

Hypothyroidism (Low Thyroid)

Things that can cause low
thyroid hormone production:[1, 2, 3, 4, 5, 6, 7, 8, 9, 10, 11, 12]

- Deficiency of zinc, copper, iodine, iron, selenium, vitamins A, B2, B3, B6, C
- Stress
- Cadmium, mercury, or lead toxicity
- Starvation
- Inadequate protein intake
- High carbohydrate diet
- Elevated cortisol
- Chronic illness
- Decreased kidney or liver function
- Medications
    Beta blockers
    Birth control pills
    Estrogen
    Lithium
    Phenytoin
    Theophylline
    Chemotherapy
- Low carbohydrate diet
- Excessive alcohol use

- Aging
- Overdose of alpha lipoic acid
- Diabetes
- Fluoride, chlorine, bromine exposure
- Pesticides
- Radiation
- Surgery
- Copper excess
- Calcium excess
- Dioxins, PCBs
- Caffeine
- Tobacco
- Foods in excess
    - Walnuts
    - Almonds
    - Sorghum
    - Peanuts
    - Pine nuts
    - Millet
    - Tapioca
    - Soy
    - Brussels sprouts
    - Cauliflower
    - Cabbage
    - Broccoli
    - Turnips
    - Mustard greens
    - Spinach
- Inadequate production of cortisol, DHEA
- Phtalates (chemicals added to plastics)
- Increased free radicals
- Fasting
- Immune system factors (IL-6, TNF-alpha, IFN-2)

Supplements:[13, 14, 15, 16, 17, 18]

Vitamin A	5,000-10,000 IU
Vitamin B3	1,000 mg
Vitamin B6	100 mg
B complex vitamins	100 mg
Vitamin B12	1,000 micrograms
Vitamin C	1,000-3,000 mg
Vitamin E	400 IU
Selenium	200 micrograms
Kelp	150 mg
L-tyrosine	1,000 mg
Vitamin D	400 IU
Zinc	25-50 mg
L-carnitine	1,000-4,000 mg
Coenzyme Q-10	30-120 mg
Magnesium	400-600 mg
Iodine	100-300 micrograms
Selenium	200-300 micrograms
GLA	240 mg
EPA/DHA	500-2,000 mg
Myrrh	20-60 mg
Sage	40-60 mg
Ashwaganda	500-1,000 mg
Milk thistle	200-300 mg
Chromium	200 micrograms
Copper	1-3 mg

47

Varicose Veins

Supplements:[1, 2, 3, 4, 5, 6]

Horse chestnut	300-600 mg
Gotu kola (Centella asiatica) 40% extract	200-400 mg
Grape seed extract	100-200 mg
Pine bark extract	50-100 mg
EPA/DHA	2,000 mg

In our office we use Vessel Max by Orthomolecular (see Appendix for availability).

48

Vegetarian

Vegetarian (Lacto-ovo)

Supplements:[1]

Carnitine	500-2,000 mg
MVI	
Vitamin B12	100 micrograms
Vitamin D	400 IU
Zinc	25 mg
Iodine	75 micrograms
Selenium	200 micrograms

Veganism

Supplements:[2]

Carnitine	500-2,000 mg
Vitamin B12	100 micrograms
Vitamin D	400 IU
Zinc	25 mg
Iron	18 mg in women pre-menopausal (blood levels thereafter)
Iodine	150 micrograms
Selenium	200 micrograms
Amino acids	2-6 per day or as prescribed by your physician
Methionine	2,000 mg (or eat brazil nuts, sesame seeds, almonds)

Weight Loss 49

Many people cannot lose weight because they are stressed. When you have excess stress, your body goes into a fight-or-flight response. Your body is getting ready to fight for survival and your blood is shunted into your organs that are essential for self-defense. Stress chemicals and hormones in your body rise: adrenaline, noradrenaline, and cortisol. Your system thinks you are not going to have time to eat because you are literally running for your life. Your body will store all the food you intake as fat so you can use it later as an energy source. *This is why you gain weight and may not be able to take it off even though you are exercising and eating right.* (See stress reduction nutrients.)

Supplements:[1, 2, 3, 4]

Vitamin E	400 IU
Selenium	100-200 micrograms
Alpha lipoic acid	100-600 mg
Coenzyme Q-10	60-200 mg
NAC	500-1,000 mg
L-carnitine	2,000-8,000 mg
CLA	3,000-4,000 mg
Chromium	200-600 micrograms
Flax seed oil	1 tablespoon
MVI	
Zinc	25 mg

Ashwaganda	200-400 mg
Siberian ginseng	100-200 mg
GLA	240-480 mg
Green tea	1-3 cups

50

Women's Health

If you are taking birth control pills or hormone replacement therapy

Supplements:[1, 2]

Inositol	1,000 mg
Magnesium	400 mg
Alpha lipoic acid	300-600 mg
L-carnitine	1,000 mg
GLA	240 mg
Phosphatidyl choline	2,000 mg
B complex	100 mg

PMS

Supplements:[3, 4, 5, 6, 7, 8, 9, 10, 11, 12, 13, 14, 15, 16, 17, 18]

Chasteberry	
Calcium	1,000-1,200 mg
Magnesium	400-800 mg
Manganese	2-5 mg
B complex	50 mg
Vitamin E	400 IU
GLA	240 mg
Vitamin A	10,000-20,000 IU
(no more than 8,000 IU if a smoker)	
Vitamin C	1,000 mg

Zinc	25-50 mg
Copper	1-2 mg
L-carnitine	500 mg
Chromium	400 micrograms
Inositol	500-1,000 mg

Painful Menstrual Cycles

Supplements:[19, 20]

B12	1,000 micrograms
EPA/DHA	2,000-3,000 mg
GLA	500-1,000 mg

Peri-Menopause Symptoms

Supplements:[21, 22]

Black cohash
Chasteberry
Dong Quai
Soy

To Prevent and Treat Cervical Dysplasia (A Precursor to Cervical Cancer)

Supplements:[23, 24]

Folic acid	800 micrograms
	(2,000-6,000 micrograms as prescription)
Vitamin C	500-1,000 mg
B complex vitamins	100 mg
Vitamin B12	1,000-5,000 micrograms
Zinc	25 mg
EPA/DHA	1,000 mg
Carotenoids	50,000-100,000 IU
	(doctor supervision required)
Vitamin E	400 IU
Selenium	200 micrograms
Indole-3-carbinol	200-400 mg

Alpha lipoic acid	100-300 mg
Quercetin	300-900 mg
Rutin	300 mg

PCOS (Polycystic Ovarian Syndrome)

Supplements:[25, 26, 27]

Inositol	12,000 mg
	(under the direction of a physician)
Chromium	600-1,000 micrograms
Zinc	25-50 mg
L-carnitine	1,000-6,000 mg
Copper	1-3 mg
Alpha lipoic acid	100-600 mg
Taurine	500-2,000 mg
B complex	50 mg
Magnesium	400-800 mg
Vitamin E	400-800 IU
Vitamin C	1,000-3,000 mg
Vitamin D	400 IU
Vanadium	50 mg
EPA/DHA	500-1,000 mg
GLA	240-480 mg

Estrogen Dominance

Supplements:[28]

Indole-3-carbinol	300-500 mg
Flax seed	1,000 mg
Soy	

Fibroid Tumors

Supplements:[29]

Natural progesterone	as prescribed by your doctor
Phosphatidyl choline	2,000 mg
Inositol	1,000 mg

Magnesium	400 mg
Alpha lipoic acid	300 mg
GLA	240-720 mg
Milk thistle	100-200 mg
L-carnitine	1,500 mg
Coenzyme Q-10	100 mg

Stop coffee

Wound Healing 51

Supplements:[1, 2, 3, 4]

Carnosine	1,000-2,000 mg
Vitamin C	2,000 mg
Arginine	1,000-3,000 mg
Pantothenic acid	100 mg

If a doctor is not a good nutritionist, he cannot be a good physician.
—Abram Hoffer, M.D., Ph.D.

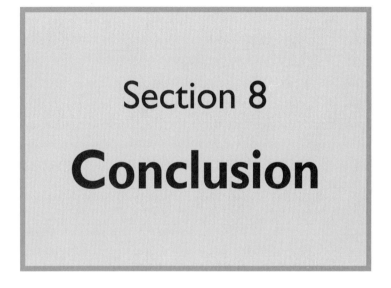

Section 8

Conclusion

The goal of this book has been to educate and to show you how nutrients can improve function to provide optimal biochemical activities in your body, thus maintaining your health and preventing disease. Medicine is at a cross roads. The role of the doctor in the near future will be to restore balances to your body, to prevent and treat chronic disease, rather than to treat an acute illness. This is called functional medicine which is an integrative, science-based healthcare approach that treats illness and promotes wellness by focusing assessment on the biochemically unique aspects of each patient, and then individually tailoring interventions to restore physiological, psychological, and structural balance.

There are seven basic principles underlying functional medicine which include the following:

- Science-based medicine that connects the emerging research base to clinical practice.
- Biochemical individuality based on genetic and environmental uniqueness.

- Patient-centered care (rather than disease-focused) which means that you are the focus of care, not the diagnosis.
- Dynamic balance of internal and external factors that affect total functioning.
- Web-like interconnections among the body's physiological processes also affect every aspect of your functionality.
- Health as a positive vitality, not merely the absence of disease.
- Promotion of organ reserve. Your heart, your lungs, your glands, and everything in your body can achieve greater stamina, better recovery from illness, and a longer "health span," not just a longer "life span."

As you have seen, this book contains a functional medicine approach to health care which focuses on understanding the fundamental physiological processes, the environmental inputs, and the genetic predispositions that influence your experience of health and disease so that interventions are focused on treating the cause of the problem, not just masking the symptoms. Changing how your system functions can have a major impact on your health. Most imbalances in functionality can be addressed; some can be completely restored to optimum function and others can be substantially improved.

This is a new age of medicine, where you the patient, are an active participant in your own treatment. Lifestyle is a very large factor. This means what you eat, how you exercise, how much stress you live with, and what nutrients you take are all elements that affect your overall health.

Ideas concerning vitamins and nutrition have changed over the years. At first vitamins were used to prevent disease, now they are used to optimize physiological function. It is now known that nutrients have numerous interactions and not just a single action as was previously believed. Up until now, RDA guidelines were used. Now optimal dosages customized to each person's own individualized needs are available. My job as a physician is not to criticize you over your lifestyle. It is to assist you in the process of optimizing your health and healing through education. It is my hope that this book has provided you with a reference for you and your health care provider to use as a framework to develop a nutritional program designed for you and you only. As your needs change, so should your vitamin program.

APPENDIX

All lab testing referenced to in this book is available through:

Great Smokies Diagnostic Laboratory
63 Zillicoa St.
Asheville, NC 28801-1074
1-800-522-4762
www.gsdl.com

Supplements from the following companies are available through your doctor, or through Binson's Home Health Care (see below) which has doctors and nurses right in the store to help you with your health care needs.

Metagenics
P.O. Box 1729
Gig Harbor, WA 98335
1-800-843-9660
www.metagenics.com

Ortho Molecular Products
3017 Business Park Drive
P.O. Box 1060
Stevens Point, WI 54481
1-800-332-2351

Designs For Health
2 North Road
East Windsor, CT 06088
1-800-847-8302
www.DesignsForHealth.com

Binson's Home Health Care Centers
26819 Lawrence Ave.
Center Line, MI 48015
1-888-BINSONS
www.binsons.com

Billie Sahley, Ph.D.
Pain & Stress Center
5282 Medical Drive, Suite 160
San Antonio, TX 78229
1-800-669-2256
www.painstresscenter.com

Life Extension
1-800-544-4440
www.LifeExtension.com

Juice Plus
National Safety Associates
4260 E. Raines Road
Memphis, Tennessee 38118
1-800-347-5947

For a compounding pharmacy near you contact:

Professional Compounding Centers of America
9901 South Wilcrest Dr.
Houston, TX 77099
1-800-331-2498
www.pccarx.com

REFERENCES

Section I

1. Murray, C., et al., "Alternative projections of mortality and disability by cause 1990-2020: global burden of disease study," *Lancet* 1997; 349:1498-1504.

2. Vita, Anthony, et al., "Aging, health risks, and cumulative disability," *NEJM* 1998; 338; 1035-41.

3. Hu, F., et al., "Diet, lifestyle, and the risk of type 2 diabetes mellitus in women," *NEJM* 2001; 345 (11): 790-797.

4. Fletcher, R., et al., "Vitamins for chronic disease prevention in adults," *JAMA* 2002; 287(23):3116.

5. Meletis, C., *Interactions Between Drugs and Natural Medicines.* Sandy, Oregon: Electric Medical Publications, 1999.

6. Fuhr, U., et al., "Drug interactions with grapefruit juice, extent, probable mechanism, and clinical relevance," *Drug Sci* 1998; 18:251-272.

7. Ibid., Meletis.

8. Colgan, M., *The New Nutrition.* Vancouver, British Columbia, Canada: Apple Publishing, 1995.

9. Lieberman, S., *The Real Vitamin and Mineral Book.* New York: Avery Publishing Group, 1997.

10. Ulene, A., *Dr. Art Ulene's Complete Guide to Vitamins, Minerals, and Herbs.* New York: Avery Publishing, 2000.

11. Ibid., Colgan, p. 14.

12. Ibid., Lieberman, p. 21.

13. Ibid., Lieberman, p. 22.

14. Bland, J., "Oxidants and antioxidants in clinical medicine: past, present, and future potential," *J. Nutr Environ Med* 1995; 5:255-280.

15. Pietrizk, K., et al., "Antioxidant, vitamins, cancer, and cardiovascular disease," *NEJM Letter to the Editor* 1996, 335(14):1065-66.

16. Krebs-Smith, S., et al., "Fruits and vegetable intakes of children and adolescents in the United States," *Arch Ped Adolesc Med* 1996; 150(1):81-86.

17. Heller, L., Seminar entitled "Healthy Women, Healthy Aging" November 15-16, 2003, p. 26.

18. Galland, L., "Person-centered diagnosis and chronic fatigue" *Metabolic Energy, Messenger Molecules, and Chronic Illness: The Functional Perspective.* Gig Harbor, Washington: Institute for Functional Medicine, 2000, p. 326.

19. Challem, J., *Syndrome X.* New York: John Wiley & Sons., Inc., 2000, p. 61.

Section 2

1. Hart, C., *The Insulin-Resistance Diet.* Chicago, Illinois: Contemporary Books, 2001, p. 91.

2. Ibid., Colgan, p.103.

3. Ibid., Liberman, p. 54.

4. Bateman, J., "Possible toxicity of herbal remedies," *Scottish Med J.* 1998; 4:7-15.

5. Ibid., Colgan, p. 104.

Chapter 1

1. Bland, J., *Clinical Nutrition: A Functional Approach.* Gig Harbor, Washington: Institute for Functional Medicine, 1999, p. 130.

2. Semba, R., et al., "Vitamin A and immunity to viral, bacterial, and protozoan infections," Proc Nutr Soc 1999; 58(3):719-27.

3. Ibid., Lieberman, *The Real Vitamin and Mineral Book*, p. 81.

4. Ibid., Bland, *Clinical Nutrition: A Functional Approach*, p. 130-131.

5. Lark, S., *The Menopause Self Help Book.* Berkeley, California: Celestial Arts, 1990, p. 101.

6. Brownstein, D., *The Miracle of Natural Hormones.* West Bloomfield, Michigan: Medical Alternatives Press, 1999; p. 135.

7. Crook, T., *The Memory Cure.* New York: Pocket Books, 1998, p. 156.

8. Ibid., Bland, *Clinical Nutrition: A Functional Approach*, p. 131.

9. Ibid., Bland, *Clinical Nutrition: A Functional Approach*, p. 131.

10. Ibid., Bland, *Clinical Nutrition: A Functional Approach*, p. 130.

11. Ibid., Bland, *Clinical Nutrition: A Functional Approach*, p. 131.

12. Ibid., Bland, *Clinical Nutrition: A Functional Approach*, p. 131.

13. Feskanich, D., et al., "Vitamin A intake and hip fracture among postmenopausal woman," *JAMA* 2002; 287(1):47-54.

14. Paran, E., et al., "Effect of lycopene, an oral natural antioxidant, on blood pressure," *J. Hypertens* 2001; 19:S74, Abstract P-1.204.

15. Paran, E., et al., "Effect of lycopene on blood pressure, serum lipoproteins, plasma homocysteine, and oxidative stress markers in grade I hypertensive patients," *Am J. Hypertens* 2001; 140-141A, Abstract P-333.

16. Ibid., Pietrizk., p. 1065-66.

Chapter 2

1. Holick, M., et al., "Vitamin D and bone health," *J. Nutr* 1996; 126:1159S-1164S.

2. Dawson-Hughes, B., et al., "Effect of vitamin D supplementation on wintertime and overall bone loss in healthy postmenopausal women," *Ann Intern Med* 1991; 115(7):505-12.

3. Dawson-Hughes, B., et al., "Effect of calcium and vitamin D supplementation on bone density in men and women 65 years of age or older," *NEJM* 1997; 337(10):670-76.

4. Collins, J., *What's Your Menopause Type?* Roseville, California: Prima Publishing, 2000, p. 207.

5. Ibid., Bland, *Clinical Nutrition: A Functional Approach*, p. 133.

6. Ibid., Bland, *Clinical Nutrition: A Functional Approach*, p. 133.

Chapter 3

1. Ibid., Bland, *Clinical Nutrition: A Functional Approach*, p. 127.

2. Meydani, S., et al., "Vitamin E supplementation and in vivo immune response in healthy elderly subjects," *JAMA* 1997; 277:1380-86.

3. Chan, A., et al., "Vitamin E and atherosclerosis," *J. Nutr* 1998; 128(10):1593-96.

4. Freedman, F., et al., "Alpha-tocopherol inhibits aggregation of human platelets by a protein kinase C-dependent mechanism," *Circulation* 1996; 94(10):2434-40.

5. Behl, C., et al., "Vitamin E protects nerve cell from amyloid and protein toxicity," *Biochem Biophys J. Res Communs* 1992; 186(2):944-50.

6. Packer, L., *The Antioxidant Miracle*. New York: John Wiley & Sons, Inc., 1999, p. 66.

7. Paolisso, G., et al., "Vitamin E improves the action of insulin," *Diabetes Care* 1989; 12:265-69.

8. Fillion, M., *Natural Prostate Healers*. Paramus, NJ: Prentice Hall Press, 1999, p. 93.

9. Ibid., Bland, *Clinical Nutrition: A Functional Approach*, p. 127.

10. Sano, M., et al., "A controlled trial of selegiline, alpha-tocopherol, or both as treatment for Alzheimer's disease. The Alzheimer's disease cooperative study," *NEJM* 1997: 336:1216-22.

11. Gaby, A., *Nutritional Therapy in Medical Practice*. Carlisle, PA: Nutrition Seminars, 2003, p. 26-7.

12. Lethem, R., et al., "Antioxidants and dementia," *Lancet* 1997; 348:1189.

13. Ibid., Crook, p. 158.

14. Ibid., Fillion, p. 93.

15. Qureshi, A., et al., "Response of hypercholesterolemic subjects to administration of tocotrienols," *Lipids* 1995; 30(12):1171-77.

16. Qureshi, A., et al., "Lowering of serum cholesterol in hypercholesterolemic humans by tocotrienols (palmvite)," *Amer Jour Clin Nutr* 1991; 53(4Suppl):1021S-1026S.

17. Tomeo, A., et al., "Antioxidant effects of tocotrienols in patients with hyperlipidemia and carotid stenosis," *Lipids* 1995; 30(12):1179-83.

Chapter 4

1. Booth, S., et al., "Skeletal functions of vitamin K-dependent proteins: not just for clotting anymore," *Nutritional Rev* 1997; 55:282-84.

2. Feskanich, D., et al., "Vitamin K intake and hip fracture in women: a prospective study, "*Am Jour Clin Nutr* 1999; 69:74-9.

3. Hidaka, T., "Treatment for patients with postmenopausal osteoporosis who have been placed on hormone replacement therapy and show a decrease in bone mineral density: effects of concomitant administration of vitamin K (2)," *J. Bone Miner Metab* 2002; 20(4):235-9.

4. Ibid., Collins, p. 211.

5. Janein, B., et al., "Low vitamin K linked to coronary calcification risk: nutritional intervention might be possible," *Family Practice News* 2002; 32(1):1-2.

6. Witteman, J., et al., "Aortic calcified plaque and cardiovascular disease (the Framingham study)," *Am J. Cardiol* 1990; 66:1060-64.

7. Ibid., Collins, p. 212.

8. "Weak bones cause heart attacks and stoke," *Collector's Edition Life Extension*, 2003.

9. Vermeer, C., et al., "A comprehensive review of vitamin K and vitamin K antagonist," *Hematol Oncol Clin North Am* 2000; 14(2):339-53.

10. Ibid., Bland, *Clinical Nutrition: A Functional Approach*, p. 136.

11. Ibid., Bland, *Clinical Nutrition: A Functional Approach*, p. 135.

Chapter 5

1. Ibid., Lark, p. 101.

2. Chan, P., et al., "Randomized double-blind, placebo-controlled study of the safety and efficacy of vitamin B complex in the treatment of nocturnal leg cramps in elderly patients with hypertension," *Jour Clin Pharm* 1998; 38(12):1151-4.

3. Ibid., Bland, *Clinical Nutrition: A Functional Approach*, p. 101.

1.1

1. Ibid., Bland, *Clinical Nutrition: A Functional Approach*, p. 105.

2. Ibid., Crook, p. 151.

3. Ibid., Crook, p. 151.

4. Ibid., Bland, *Clinical Nutrition: A Functional Approach*, p. 106.

5. Ibid., Crook p. 152.

6. Ibid., Bland, *Clinical Nutrition: A Functional Approach*, p. 105.

7. Ibid., Colgan, p. 79.

8. Ibid., Bland, *Clinical Nutrition: A Functional Approach*, p. 106.

9. Ibid., Gaby, *Nutritional Therapy in Medical Practice*, p. 6.

1.2

1. Ibid., Collins, p. 194.

2. Ibid., Bland, *Clinical Nutrition: A Functional Approach*, p. 108.

3. Ibid., Bland, *Clinical Nutrition: A Functional Approach*, p. 107

4. Ibid., Gaby, *Nutritional Therapy in Medical Practice*, p. 7.

5. Ibid., Bland, *Clinical Nutrition: A Functional Approach*, p. 108.

6. Ibid., Colgan, p. 89.

7. Schoenen, J., et al., "High-dose riboflavin as a prophylactic treatment of migraine: results of an open pilot study," *Cephalgia* 1994; 14(5):328-9.

8. Ibid., Bland, *Clinical Nutrition: A Functional Approach*, p. 108.

1.3

1. Ibid., Bland, *Clinical Nutrition: A Functional Approach*, p. 110.

2. DiPalma, J., et al., "Use of niacin as a drug," *Annu Rev Nutr* 1991; 11:169-87.

3. Polo, V., et al., "Nicotinamide improves nsulin secretion and metabolic control in lean type 2 diabetic patients with secondary failure to sulphonylureas," *Acta Diabetol* 1998; 35(1):61-4.

4. Ibid., Bland, *Clinical Nutrition: A Functional Approach*, p. 111.

5. Ibid., Bland, *Clinical Nutrition: A Functional Approach*, p. 110.

6. Ibid., Collins, p. 195.

7. Gang, R., et al., "Niacin treatment increases plasma homocysteine levels," *Am Heart Jour* 1999; 138(6 Pt. 1):1082-7.

8. Ibid., Gaby, *Nutritional Therapy in Medical Practice*, p. 8.

9. Ibid., Bland, *Clinical Nutrition: A Functional Approach*, p. 110.

10. Ibid., Gaby, *Nutritional Therapy in Medical Practice*, p. 7-8.

1.4

1. Ibid., Bland, *Clinical Nutrition: A Functional Medicine Approach*, p. 112.

2. Ibid., Bland, *Clinical Nutrition: A Functional Medicine Approach*, p. 112.

3. Schwaberdal, P., et al., "Pantothenic acid deficiency as a factor contributing to the development of hypertension," *Cardiology* 1985; 72(Suppl 1):187-89.

4. Goldman, R., *Human Growth Factors*. Chicago: American Academy of Anti-Aging Physicians, 2003, p. 50-51.

5. Ibid., Crook, p. 153.

6. Ibid., Bland, *Clinical Nutrition: A Functional Approach*, p. 112.

7. Ibid., Bland, *Clinical Nutrition: A Functional Approach*, p. 112.

8. Ibid., Berkson, p. 55.

1.5

1. Ibid., Bland, *Clinical Nutrition: A Functional Approach*, p. 113.

2. Ibid., Bland, *Clinical Nutrition: A Functional Approach*, p. 115.

3. Schmidt, M., *Tired of Being Tired*. Berkeley, Calfornia: Frog, Ltd., 1995, p. 62.

4. Ibid., Crook, p. 154.

5. Ibid., Collins, p. 196.

6. Ibid., Bland, *Clinical Nutrition: A Functional Approach*, p. 115.

7. Ibid., Gaby, *Nutritional Therapy in Medical Practice*, p. 15.

8. Perlmutter, D., "The brain on fire: the role of inflammation in neurodegenerative disorders," A4M Conference 2003, p. 174.

9. Ibid., Bland, *Clinical Nutrition: A Functional Approach*, p. 114.

10. Schaumberg, H., et al., "Sensory neuropathy from pyridoxine abuse: a new megavitamin syndrome," *NEJM* 1983; 309:445-448.

11. Ibid., Bland, *Clinical Nutrition: A Functional Approach*, p. 115.

12. Ibid., Bland, *Clinical Nutrition: A Functional Approach*, p. 114.

13. Ibid., Gaby, *Nutritional Therapy in Medical Practice*, p. 13-14.

1.6

1. Ibid., Bland, *Clinical Nutrition: A Functional Approach*, p.116.

2. Ibid., Bland, *Clinical Nutrition: A Functional Approach*, p. 116.

3. Ibid., Collins, p. 199.

4. Miller, A., et al., "Homocysteine metabolism: nutritional modulation and impact on health and disease," *Alt Med Rev* 1997; 2(4):234-254.

5. VanGoor, V., et al., "B12 deficiency and mental impairment," *Review: Age and Ageing* 1995; 24:536-42.

6. Ibid., Schmidt, p. 64.

7. Ibid., Gaby, *Nutritional Therapy in Medical Practice*, p. 18.

8. Ibid., Gaby, *Nutritional Therapy in Medical Practice*, p. 18.

9. Ibid., Perlmutter, "The brain on fire: the role of inflammation in neurodegenerative disorders," p. 174.

10. Ibid., Bland, *Clinical Nutrition: A Functional Approach*, p. 117.

11. Ibid., Bland, *Clinical Nutrition: A Functional Approach*, p. 117.

12. Ibid., Gaby, Nutritional Therapy in Medical Practice, p. 16-17.

13. Boltiglieri, T., et al., "Folate, vitamin B12, neuropsychiatric disorders," *Nutr Rev* 1996; 54(2):138-42.

1.7

1. Hochman, L., et al., "Brittle nails: response to daily biotin supplementation," *Cutis* 1993; 51(4):303-5.

2. Maebashi, M., et al., "Therapeutic evaluation of the effect of biotin on hyperglycemia patients with non-insulin dependant diabetes mellitus," *Journ of Clin Biochem and Nutri* 1993; 14:211-18.

3. Ibid., Bland, *Clinical Nutrition: A Functional Approach*, p. 122.

4. Ibid., Bland, *Clinical Nutrition: A Functional Approach*, p. 121.

5. Ibid., Bland, *Clinical Nutrition: A Functional Approach*, p. 121.

6. Ibid., Gaby, *Nutritional Therapy in Medical Practice*, p. 16.

7. Ibid., Bland, *Clinical Nutrition: A Functional Approach*, p. 122.

8. Shang, H., et al., "A high biotin diet improves the impaired glucose tolerance of long-term spontaneously hyperglycemic rats with non-insulin-dependent diabetes mellitus," *J. Nutr Sci Vitamins* 1996; 42:517-26.

9. Koutsilos, D., et al., "Biotin for diabetic peripheral neuropathy," *Biomed Phamacother* 1990; 44(10):511-4.

10. Coggeshall, J., et al., "Biotin status and plasma glucose in diabetes," *Ann NY Acad Sci* 1985; 447:389.

11. Ibid., Gaby, *Nutritional Therapy in Medical Practice*, p. 15-16.

1.8

1. Crayhon, R., "Aging well in the 21st century," Seminar 2002, p. 15.

2. Ibid., Crayhon, "Aging well in the 21st century," p. 15.

3. Ibid., Crayhon, "Aging well in the 21st century," p. 16.

4. Ibid., Crayhon, "Aging well in the 21st century," p. 15.

5. Benjamin, J., et al., "Double-blind, placebo-controlled, crossover trial of inositol treatment for panic disorder," *Am J Psychiatry* 1995; 152:1084-86.

6. Sundkvist, G., et al., "Sorbitol and myo-inositol levels and morphology of neural nerve in relation to peripheral nerve function and clinical neuropathy in men with diabetic, impaired, and normal glucose tolerance," *Diabetic Med* 2000; 17:259-268.

7. Levine, J., et al., "Combination of inositol and serotonin reuptake inhibitors in the treatment of depression," *Biol Psychiatry* 1999; 45(3):270-3.

1.9

1. Ibid., Bland, *Clinical Nutrition: A Functional Approach*, p. 119.

2. Bland, J., "Nutrients as Biological Response Modifiers," *Applying Functional Medicine in Clinical Practice*. Gig Harbor, Washington: Functional Medicine Institute, 2002 p. 48.

3. Weler, M., et al., "Periconceptional folic acid exposure and risk of occurrent neural tube defects," *JAMA* 1993; 269:1257-1261.

4. Kwasniewska, A., et al., "Folate deficiency and cervical intraepithelial neoplasia," *Eur J Gynaecol Oncol* 1997; 18(6):526-30.

5. Butterworth, C., et al., "Folate deficiency and cervical dysplasia," *JAMA* 1992; 267(4):528-33.

6. Ibid., Collins, p. 201.

7. Ibid., Collins, p. 201.

8. Ibid., Collins, p. 201.

9. Ibid., Bland, *Clinical Nutrition: A Functional Approach*, p. 120.

10. Ibid., Bland, *Disorders of the Brain: Emerging Therapies in Complex Neurologic and Psychiatric Conditions*, p. 50.

11. Ibid., Bland, *Clinical Nutrition: A Functional Approach*, p. 119.

12. Ibid., Perlmutter, "The Brain on fire: the role of inflammation in neurodegenerative disorders," p. 174.

13. Ibid., Goldman, *Human Growth Factors*, p. 55.

14. Ibid., Bland, *Clinical Nutrition: A Functional Approach*, p. 119.

15. Ibid., Bland, *Clinical Nutrition: A Functional Approach*, p. 121.

16. Ibid., Gaby, *Nutritional Therapy in Medical Practice*, p. 10.

Chapter 6

1. Ibid., Bland, *Clinical Nutrition: A Functional Approach*, p. 124.

2. Ibid., Collins, p. 203.

3. Ibid., Berkson, p. 86.

4. Perlmutter, D., *BrainRecovery.com*. Naples, Florida: The Perlmutter Health Center, 2000, p. 28.

5. Houston, M., *What Your Doctor May Not Tell You About Hypertension*. New York: Warner Books, Inc., 2003, p. 67.

6. Debusk, R., et al., "Dietary supplements and cardiovascular disease," *Curr Atheroscler Rep* 2000; 2:508-514.

7. Feldman, E., et al., "The role of vitamin C and antioxidants in hypertension," *Nutrition and the M.D* 1998; 24:1-4.

8. Trout, D., et al., "Vitamin C and cardiovascular risk factors," *Am J Clin Nutr* 1991; 53:322-25.

9. Fotherby, M., et al., "Effect of vitamin C on ambulatory blood pressure and plasma lipids in older persons," *J. Hypertens* 2000; 18; 411-415.

10. Simon, J., et al., "Vitamin C and cardiovascular disease a review," *J. Amer Coll Nutr* 1992; 11:107-125.

11. Block, G., et al., "Ascorbic acid status and subsequent diastolic and systolic blood pressure," *Hypertension* 2001; 37:261-67.

12. Ibid., Bland, *Clinical Nutrition: A Functional Approach*, p. 125.

13. Sinatra, S., "Alternative interventions for preventing and treating cardiovascular disease," A4M conference June 2003, p. 92.

14. Ibid., Fillion, p. 182.

15. Ibid., Bland, *Clinical Nutrition: A Functional Approach*, p. 124.

16. Ibid., Colgan, p. 84.

17. Ibid., Bland, *Clinical Nutrition: A Functional Approach*, p. 125.

18. Ibid., Bland, *Clinical Nutrition: A Functional Approach*, p. 125.

19. Ibid., Packer, p. 78.

Section 3

Chapter 1

1. Ibid., Bland, *Clinical Nutrition: A Functional Approach*, p. 147-48.

2. Ibid., Bland, *Clinical Nutrition: A Functional Approach*, p. 147.

3. Ibid., Bland, *Clinical Nutrition: A Functional Approach*, p. 147.

4. Nguyen, U., et al., "Aspartame ingestion increases urinary, calcium, but not oxalate excretion, in healthy subjects," *J. Clin Endocrinol Metab* 1998; 83(1):165-168.

5. Ibid., Crook, p. 159.

6. Ibid., Colgan, p. 65.

7. Germano, R., *The Osteoporosis Solution*, New York: Kensington Publishing Corp., 1999, p. 102.

8. Nachtigall, L, *Estrogen The Facts Can Change Your Life*. New York: HarperCollins, p. 154.

9. Ibid., Crook, p. 159.

10. Smith, P, *HRT: The Answers*. Traverse City, MI: Healthy Living Books, 2003, p. 65.

11. Ibid., Colgan, p. 66.

12. Ibid., Bland, *Clinical Nutrition: A Functional Approach*, p. 148.

13. Ibid., Colgan, p. 63.

14. Ibid., Smith, p. 64.

15. Ibid., Smith, p. 49.

16. Ibid., Smith, p. 63-64.

17. Ibid., Germano, p. 103.

18. Ibid., Germano, p. 101.

20. Ibid., Colgan, p. 101.

21. Ibid., Gaby, *Nutritional Therapy in Medical Practice*, p. 32

22. Ibid., Gaby, *Nutritional Therapy in Medical Practice*, p. 33.

Chapter 2

1. Ibid., Bland, *Clinical Nutrition: A Functional Approach*, p. 153-155.

2. Yang, C., et al., "Calcium and magnesium in drinking water and risk from cardiovascular disease," *Stroke* 1998; 29(2):411-14.

3. Paolisso, G., et al., "Improved insulin response and action by chronic magnesium administration in aged NIDDM subjects," *Diabetes Care* 1989; 12(4):265-72.

4. Braverman, E., *Hypertension and Nutrition* New Cannan, Conn: Keats Publishing, Inc. 1996, p. 152.

5. Ibid., Braverman, p. 151.

6. Ibid., Braverman, p. 151.

7. Ibid., Braverman, p. 151.

8. Davis, W., et al., "Monotherapy with magnesium increases abonormally low HDL cholesterol:A clinical assay," *Curr Ther Res.* 1984; 36:341-46.

9. Gaby, A. *Magnesium*. New Canaan, Conn: Keats Publishing, 1994, p. 38.

10. Galland, L, "Magnesium and immune function: an overview," *Magnesium* 1988; 7:290-99.

11. Ibid., Bland, *Clinical Nutrition: A Functional Approach*, p. 155.

12. Ibid., Gaby, *Magnesium*, p. 34.

13. Simontacchi, C., *The Crazy Makers*. New York: Jeremy P. Tarcher/Putnam, 2000, p. 112.

14. Doghlan, H., et al., "Magnesium in mitral valve prolapse syndrome," *Magnesium Trace Elem* 1990; 9:319-320.

15. Ibid., Bland, *Clinical Nutrition: A Functional Approach*, p. 156.

16. Ramadan, W., et al., "Low brain magnesium in migraine," *Headache* 1989; 29:590-93.

17. Faccinetti, F., et al., "Magnesium prohylaxis of menstrual migraine: effects on intracellular magnesium," *Headache* 1991; 31:298-304.

18. Weaver, K., et al., "Magnesium and migraine," *Headache* 1990; 30:168.

19. Ibid., Crook, p. 160-161.

20. Ibid., Gaby, *Nutritional Therapy in Medical Practice*, p. 36.

21. Ibid., Crook, p. 160.

22. Ibid., Bland, *Clinical Nutrition: A Functional Approach*, p. 154.

23. Ibid., Bland, *Clinical Nutrition: A Functional Approach*, p. 156.

24. Ibid., Gaby, *Nutritional Therapy in Medical Practice*, p. 34-35.

Chapter 3

1. Ibid., Bland, *Clinical Nutrition: A Functional Approach*, p. 151.

2. Ibid., Bland, *Clinical Nutrition: A Functional Approach*, p. 153.

3. Ibid., Bland, *Clinical Nutrition: A Functional Approach*, p. 152.

Chapter 4

1. Ibid., Bland, *Clinical Nutrition: A Functional Approach*, p. 159.

2. Ibid., Bland, *Clinical Nutrition: A Functional Approach*, p. 158.

3. Ibid., Bland, *Clinical Nutrition: A Functional Approach*, p. 157.

4. Ibid., Bland, *Clinical Nutrition: A Functional Approach*, p. 160.

5. Ibid., Bland, *Clinical Nutrition: A Functional Approach*, p. 160.

6. Ibid., Bland, *Clinical Nutrition: A Functional Approach*, p. 158.

7. Ibid., Gaby, *Nutritional Therapy in Medical Practice*, p. 37.

Chapter 5

1. Newnhau, R., et al., "Essentiality of boron for healthy bones and joints," *Environ Health Perspect* 1994; 102 (Suppl)7:83-5.

2. Ibid., Bland, *Clinical Nutrition: A Functional Approach*, p. 182.

3. Zhang, Z., et al., "Boron is associated with decreased risk of prostate cancer," *FASEB J.* 2001; 1:394-7.

4. Hunt, C., et al., "Dietary boron as a physiological regulator of the normal inflammatory response: a review and current research progress," *J. Trace Elem Med* 1999; 12:221-33.

5. Penland, J., et al., "The importance of boron nutrition for brain and psychological function," *Biol Trac Elem Res* 1998; 66:299-317.

6. Penland, J., et al., "Dietary boron, brain function, and cognitive performance," *Environ Health Perspect* 1994; 102(Suppl)7:65-72.

7. Ibid., Bland, *Clinical Nutrition: A Functional Approach*, p. 183.

8. Ibid., Colgan, p. 97.

Chapter 6

1. Evans, G., *Chromium Picolinate*. New York: Avery Publishing Group, 1996.

2. Ibid., Evans, p. 3.

3. Ibid., Bland, *Clinical Nutrition: A Functional Approach*, p. 161.

4. Press, R., et al., "The effect of chromium picolinate on serum cholesterol and apoliporotein fractions in human subjects," *Western J. of Med* 1990; 152:41-45.

5. Preuss, H., et al., "Chromium update: examining recent literature 1997-1998," *Curr Opin Clin Nutr Metab Care* 1998; 1:509-12.

6. Ibid., Evans, p. 3.

7. Bahadori, B., et al., "Treatment with chromium picolinate improves lean body mass in patients following weight reduction," *Inter Journ of Obesity* 1995; 19(Suppl 12):38.

8. Crayhon, R., *Robert Crayhon's Nutrition Made Simple*. New York: M. Evans and Company, 1994, p. 123.

9. Ibid., Liberman, p. 168.

10. Ibid., Bland, "Nutrients as Biological Response Markers," p. 33.

11. Ibid., Bland, *Clinical Nutrition: A Functional Approach*, p. 161.

12. Ibid., Evans, p. 72.

13. Ibid., Bland, *Clinical Nutrition: A Functional Approach*, p. 161.

14, Ibid., Evans, p. 72.

15. Anderson, R., et al., "Effect of chromium supplementation on Cr excretion of human subjects and correlation of Cr excretion with selected clinical parameters," *Jour of Nurt* 1983; 113:276-281.

16. Ibid., Bland, *Clinical Nutrition: A Functional Approach*, p. 162.

Chapter 7

1. Ibid., Bland, "Nutrients as Biological Response Modifiers," p. 34

2. Ibid., Bland, "Nutrients as Biological Response Modifiers," p. 35.

3. Ibid., Bland, *Clinical Nutrition: A Functional Approach*, p. 165, 167.

4. Ibid., Gaby, *Nutritional Therapy in Medical Practice*, p. 41.

5. Ibid., Bland, *Clinical Nutrition: A Functional Approach*, p. 166.

6. Ibid., Bland, *Clinical Nutrition: A Functional Approach*, p. 166.

7. Ibid., Bland, *Clinical Nutrition: A Functional Approach*, p. 167.

8. Ibid., Gaby, *Nutritional Therapy in Medical Practice*, p. 41.

Chapter 8

1. Ibid., Bland, *Clinical Nutrition: A Functional Approach*, p. 169.

2. Ibid., Lark, p. 105.

3. Ibid., Goldman, *Human Growth Factors*, p. 60.

4. Ibid., Bland, *Clinical Nutrition: A Functional Approach*, p. 169.

5. Ibid., Bland, *Clinical Nutrition: A Functional Approach*, p. 169.

6. Ibid., Bland, *Clinical Nutrition: A Functional Approach*, p. 169.

Chapter 9

1. Ibid., Bland, "Nutrients as Biological Response Modifiers," p. 35.

2. Ibid., Simontacchi, p. 114.

3. Ibid., Bland, *Clinical Nutrition: A Functional Approach*, p. 173.

4. Ibid., Gaby, *Nutritional Therapy in Medical Practice*, p. 42.

5. Ibid., Bland, *Clinical Nutrition: A Functional Approach*, p. 170.

6. Ibid., Gaby, *Nutritional Therapy in Medical Practice*, p. 42.

7. Ibid., Bland, *Clinical Nutrition: A Functional Approach*, p. 170.

8. Ibid., Bland, *Clinical Nutrition: A Functional Approach*, p. 172.

9. Ibid., Gaby, *Nutritional Therapy in Medical Practice*, p. 42.

10. Ibid., Gaby, *Nutritional Therapy in Medical Practice*, p. 42.

Chapter 10

1. Ibid., Bland, *Clinical Nutrition: A Functional Approach*, p. 174.

2. Ibid., Bland, "Nutrients as Biological Response Modifiers," p. 35.

3. Ibid., Bland, *Clinical Nutrition: A Functional Approach*, p. 175.

4. Ibid., Bland, *Clinical Nutrition: A Functional Approach* p. 179.

5. Ibid., Gaby, *Nutritional Therapy in Medical Practice*, p. 36.

6. Ibid., Bland, "Nutrients as Biological Response Modifiers," p. 35.

7. Ibid., Bland, *Clinical Nutrition: A Functional Approach*, p. 175.

Chapter 11

1. Ibid., Bland, *Clinical Nutrition: A Functional Approach*, p. 176.

2. Ibid., Bland, *Clinical Nutrition: A Functional Approach*, p. 177.

3. Ibid., Bland, *Clinical Nutrition: A Functional Approach*, p. 177.

4. Ibid., Colgan, p. 98.

5. Ibid., Gaby, *Nutritional Therapy in Medical Practice*, p. 46.

Chapter 12

1. Ibid., Packer, p. 143.

2. Ibid., Packer, p. 143.

3. Ibid., Bland, *Clinical Nutrition: A Functional Approach*, p, 178.

4. Ibid., Bland, *Clinical Nutrition: A Functional Approach*, p. 180.

5. Ibid., Berkson, p. 89.

6. Ibid., Bland, *Clinical Nutrition: A Functional Approach*, p. 179.

7. Ibid., Fillion, p. 221.

Chapter 14

1. Goldfine, A., et al., "Vanadium improves insulin sensitivity," *J. Clin Endocrinol Metabol* 1995; 80(11):3311-19.

2. Ibid., Bland, *Clinical Nutrition: A Functional Approach*, p. 181.

3. Ibid., Bland, *Clinical Nutrition: A Functional Approach*, p. 182.

4. Ibid., Bland, *Clinical Nutrition: A Functional Approach*, p.182.

Chapter 15

1. Ibid., Bland, "Nutrients as biological response modifiers," p. 31.

2. Ibid., Fillion, p. 90.

3. Ibid., Bland, "Nutrients as biological response modifiers," p. 31.

4. Ibid., Schmidt, *Tired of Being Tired*, p. 67.

5. Ibid., Goldman, *Human Growth Factors*, p. 58.

6. Ibid., Bland, "Nutrients as biological response modifiers," p. 32.

7. Ibid., Bland, *Clinical Nutrition: A Functional Approach*, p. 163.

8. Ibid., Fillion, p. 90.

9. Ibid., Bland, "Nutrients as biological response modifiers," p. 31.

10. Ibid., Bland, *Clinical Nutrition: A Functional Approach*, p. 164.

11. Ibid., Gaby, *Nutritional Therapy in Medical Practice*, p. 40.

12. Ibid., Fillion, p. 205.

13. Ibid., Gaby, *Nutritional Therapy in Medical Practice*, p. 38-40.

Section 4

1. Lerman, R., "Nutrients as biological response modifiers: fatty acids and inflammation," *Applying Functional Medicine in Clinical Practice*. Gig Harbor, Washington: Institute for Functional Medicine, 2002, p. 33.

2. Schmidt, M., *Brain-Building Nutrition: The Healing Power of Fats and Oils*.

Berkeley, CA: Frog, Ltd., 2001.

3. Erasmus, Udo, *Fats that Heal, Fats that Kill*. Burnaby, BC, Canada: Alive Books,

1993.

4. Ibid., Colgan, p. 146-149.

5. Ibid., Bland, *Clinical Nutrition: A Functional Approach*, p. 71-95.

6. Lerman, R., "The essential fatty acids in psychiatric and neurological dysfunction," *Brain Biochemistry and Nutrition*. Gig Harbor Washington: Institute for Functional Medicine, 2002, p. 65.

7. Goodman, J., *The Omega Solution*. Roseville, CA: Prima Publishing, 2001, p. 47.

8. Ibid., Goodman, p. 51.

9. Ibid., Bland, *Clinical Nutrition: A Functional Approach*, p. 279.

10. Ibid., Lerman, "Nutrients as biological response modifiers," p. 1.

11. Holman, R., et al. "The slow discovery of the importance of w3 essential fatty acids in human health," *J. Nutr* 1998; 128:427S-433S.

12. Siguel, E., et al., "Prevalence of essential fatty acid deficiency in patients with chronic gastrointestinal disorders," *Metabolism* 1996; 45(1):12-23.

13. Belluzzi, A., et al., "Polyunsaturated fatty acids and inflammatory bowel disease," *Am J Clin Nutr* 2000; 71(1):339S-342S.

14. Oliver, M., et al., "Diet and coronary disease," *Br Med Bull* 1981; 37:49-58.

15. Connor, S., et al., "Are fish oils beneficial in the prevention and treatment of coronary artery disease?" *Am J Clin Nutr* 1997; 66(4 Suppl):1020S-1031S.

16. Kris-Etherton, P., et al., "American Heart Association Nutrition Committee : Fish consumption, fish oil, omega 3 fatty acids and cardiovascular disease," *Circulation* 2002; 106:2747-57.

17. Hu, F., et al., "Fish and omega 3 fatty acid intake and risk of coronary heart disease in women," *JAMA* 2002; 287(14):1815-21.

18. Bucher, H., et al., "N-3 polyunsaturated fatty acid in coronary heart disease: a meta-analysis of random-controlled trials," *Am J Med* 2002; 112(4)298-304.

19. Tiemeier, H., et al., "Plasma fatty acid composition and depression are associated in the elderly: the Rotterdam study," *Am J. Clin Nutr* 2003; 78(1):40-46.

20. Marangell, L., "A double-blind, placebo-controlled study of the omega-3-fatty acid docosahexanoic acid in the treatment of major depression," *Am J Psychiatry* 2003; 160(3):996-98.

21. Mischoulov, D., et al., "Docosahexanoic acid and omega-3-fatty acids in depression." *Psychiatr Clin North Am* 2000; 4:785-94.

22. Kremer, J., et al., "N-3 fatty acid supplements in rheumatoid arthritis," *Am J Clin Nutr* 2000; 71(1Suppl):349S-351S.

23. Ibid., Gaby, *Nutritional Therapy in Medical Practice*, p. 29-31.

24. Ornish, D., et al., "Intensive lifestyle changes for reversal of coronary heart disease." *JAMA* 1998; 280(23):2001-07.

25. Vognild, E., et al., "Effects of dietary marine oils and olive oil on fatty acid composition, platelet membrane fluidity, platelet responses, and serum lipids in healthy humans," *Lipids* 1998; 3(4):3427-36.

26. Stevens, L., et al., "Essential fatty acid metabolism in boys with attention-deficit hyperactivity disorder," *Am J Clin Nutr* 1995; 62:762-8.

27. Lorenz, R., et al., "Supplementation with N-3 fatty acid from fish oil in chronic irritable bowel disease: A random, placebo-controlled, double-blind, cross-over trial," *J. Intern Med Suppl* 1989; 225(731):225-32.

28. Kang, J., et al., "Prevention of fatal cardiac arrhythmias by polyunsaturated fatty acids," *Amer J Clin Nutr* 2000; 71(1Suppl):2025-75.

29. Harris, W., et al., "Omega-e-fatty acids and serum lipoproteins: human studies," *Am J Clin Nutr* 1997; 65:1645S-1654S.

30. Geusens, P., et al., "Long-term effect of omega-3 fatty acid supplementation in active rheumatoid arthritis—a 12-month, double-blind, controlled study," *Arthritis and Rheumatism* 1996; 37(6):824-29.

31. Mayser, P., et al., "Omega-3 fatty acid-based lipid infusion in patients with chronic plaque psoriasis: results of a double-blind, randomized, placebo-controlled, multicenter trial," *Jour Am Academ Of Derm* 1998; 38:539-47.

32. Watanabe, T., et al., "The effect of a newly developed ointment containing eicosapentaenoic acid and docosahexaenoic acid in the treatment of atopic dermatitis," *J. Med Inves* 1999; 46: 173-77.

33. Bates, D., et al., "A double-blind controlled trial of long-chain omega-3 polyunsaturated fatty acids in the treatment of multiple sclerosis," *J. Neurol, Neurosurg, Psych* 1989; 52: 18-22.

34. Nordvik., I., et al., "Effect of dietary advice and omega-3 supplementation in newly diagnosed MS patient," *Acta Neurol Scandia* 2000; 102(3):143-49.

35. Ibid., Goodman, p. 182.

36. Ibid., Goodman, p. 175.

37. Ibid., Perlmutter, *BrainRecovery.com*, p. 109.

38. Ibid., Perlmutter, *BrainRecovery.com*, p. 48.

39. Kalmijn, S., et al., "Fatty acid intake and the risk of dementia and cognitive decline; a review of clnical and epidemiological studies," *J. Nutr Health Aging* 2000; 4(4):202-7.

40. Kallmijn, S. et al., "Polyunsaturated fatty acids, antioxidants, and cognitive function in very old men," *Am J Epidemiol* 1997; 145(1):33-41.

41. Stenson, W., et al. "Dietary supplementation with fish oil in ulcerative colitis," *Ann of Int Med* 1992; 116:609-14.

42. Laugharne, J., et al., "Fatty acids ad schizophrenia," *Lipids* 1996; 31(S):S163-65.

43. Ibid., Schmidt, Brain-Building Nutrition, p. 13.

44. Ibid., Schmidt, Brain-Building Nutrition, p. 76.

45. Ibid., Colgan, p. 144.

46. Ibid., Colgan, p. 145.

47. Ibid., p. 145.

48. Ibid., p. 145.

Section 5

1. Sahley, B. *Heal with Amino Acids and Nutrients*. San Antonio Texas: Pain & Stress Publications, 2000.

2. Sahley, B., *Control Hyperactivity, ADD Naturally*. San Antonio, Texas: Pain & Stress Publications, 1999, p. 44

Chapter 1

1. Ibid., Sahley, *Heal with Amino Acids*, p. 23.

2. Ibid., Sahley, *Heal with Amino Acids*, p. 23.

Chapter 2

1. Klatz, R., *The New Anti-Aging Revolution*. North Bergen, New Jersey: Basic Health Publications, 2003, p. 231.

2. Sinatra, S., *Heart Sense For Women*. Washington, DC: LifeLine Press, 2000, p. 150.

3. Efron, D., et al., "Role of arginine in immunonutrition," *J. Gastroenterol* 2000; 35(suppl 12):20-3.

4. Ibid., Sahley, *Heal with Amino Acids*, p. 23-24.

5. Siani, A., et al., "Blood pressure and metabolic changes during dietary L-arginine supplementation in human," *Am J. Hypertens* 2000; 13(5, Pt.1):547-51.

6. Ibid., Sahley, *Heal with Amino Acids*, p. 25.

7. Ibid., Klatz, *The New Anti-Aging Revolution*, p. 231.

8. Great Smokies Diagnostic Laboratory Interpretive Guidelines for Amino Acid Analysis.

Chapter 3

1. Ibid., Sahley, *Heal with Amino Acids*, p. 25.

2. Ibid., Sahley, *Heal with Amino Acids*, p. 26.

Chapter 4

1. Ibid., Klatz, *The New Anti-Aging Revolution*, p. 235.

2. Ibid., Klatz, *The New Anti-Aging Revolution*, p. 235.

3. Ibid., Klatz, *The New Anti-Aging Revolution*, p. 236.

4. Ibid., Gaby, *Nutritional Therapy in Medical Practice*, p. 63.

5. Ibid., Sahley, *Heal with Amino Acids*, p. 32.

6. Ibid., Gaby, *Nutritional Therapy in Medical Practice*, p. 63.

Chapter 5

1. Shabert, J., *The Ultimate Nutrient Glutamine*. Garden City Park, New York: Avery Publishing Group, 1994, p. 2.

2. Maskovitz, B., et al., "Glutamine metabolism and utilization: relevance to major problems in health care," *Pharmacol Res* 1994; 30(1):61-71.

3. Ibid., Sahley, *Heal with Amino Acids.*, p. 35-37.

4. Ibid., Klatz, *The New Anti-Aging Revolution*, p. 238.

5. Keast, D., et al., "Depression of plasma glutamine concentration after exercise stress and its possible influence on the immune system," *Med J. Aust* 1995; 162(1):15-8.

6. Nurjhan, N., et al., "Glutamine: a major gluconeogenic precursor and vehicle for interorgan carbon transport in man," *Jour Clin Invest* 1995; 95(1):272-7.

7. Peck., L., et al., "Glutamine should be figured into inflammatory bowel disease formulations," *Family Practice News* 1994; June, p; 22.

8. Welbourne, T., et al., "Increased plasma bicarbonate and growth hormone after an oral glutamine load," *Amer Jour Clin Nutr* 1995; 61(5):1058-61.

9. Ibid., Klatz, *The New Anti-Aging Revolution*, p. 238.

10. Ibid., Klatz, *The New Anti-Aging Revolution*, p. 240.

Chapter 6

1. Ibid., Klatz., *The New Anti-Aging Revolution*, p. 241.

2. Ibid., Sahley, *Heal with Amino Acids*, p. 40.

3. Ibid., Sahley, *Heal with Amino Acids*, p. 40.

4. Ibid., Klatz, *The New Anti-Aging Revolution*, p. 242.

Chapter 7

1. Ibid., Sahley, *Heal with Amino Acids*, p. 40.

2. Ibid., Klatz, *The New Anti-Aging Revolution*, p. 243.

3. Ibid., *Great Smokies Interpretive Guidelines*.

Chapter 8

1. Ibid., Klatz, *The New Anti-Aging Revolution*, p. 244.

2. Ibid., Sahley, *Heal with Amino Acids*, p. 41.

3. Ibid., Sahley, *Heal with Amino Acids*, p. 41.

4. Ibid., Klatz, *The New Anti-Aging Revolution*, p. 245.

5. Ibid., Klatz, *The New Anti-Aging Revolution*, p. 244.

6. Ibid., Great Smokies Interpretive Guidelines.

7. Ibid., Klatz, *The New Anti-Aging Revolution*, p. 245.

Chapter 9

1. Ibid., Klatz, *The New Anti-Aging Revolution*, p. 246.

2. Ibid., Sahley, *Heal with Amino Acids*, p. 41-42.

3. Ibid., Klatz, *The New Anti-Aging Revolution*, p. 246.

4. Ibid., Sahley, *Heal with Amino Acids*, p. 42.

Chapter 10

1. Ibid., Sahley, *Heal with Amino Acids*, p. 45.

2. Ibid., Klatz, *The New Anti-Aging Revolution*, p. 248.

3. Ibid., Klatz, *The New Anti-Aging Revolution*, p. 248.

4. Ibid., Klatz, *The New Anti-Aging Revolution*, p. 248.

5. Ibid., *Great Smokies Interpretive Guidelines*.

Chapter 11

1. Ibid., Sahley, *Heal with Amino Acids.*, p. 45.

Chapter 12

1. Ibid., Sahley, *Heal with Amino Acids.*, p. 45.

2. Ibid., Klatz, *The New Anti-Aging Revolution*, p. 250.

Chapter 13

1. Ibid., Klatz, *The New Anti-Aging Revolution*, p. 252-253.

2. Ibid., Sahley, *Heal with Amino Acids*, p. 48.

3. Kendler, B., et al., "Taurine: an overview of its role in preventive medicine," *Prev Med* 1989; 18(1):70-100.

4. Huxtable, R., et al. "Physiologic actions of taurine," *Physiol Rev* 1992; 72:101-163.

5. Ibid., Goldman, *Human Growth Factors*, p. 69.

6. Chapman, R., et al., "Taurine and the heart," *Cardiovasc Res* 1993; 27(3):358-63.

7. Redmond, H., et al., "Immunonutrition: the role of taurine," *Nutrition* 1998; 14(7-8):599-604.

8. Ibid., Crayhon, "Aging well in the 21st century," 2002.

9. Ibid., Gaby, *Nutritional Therapy in Medical Practice*, p. 58.

10. Dawson, R., "An Age-related decline in striatal taurine is correlated with a loss of dopaminergic markers," *Brain Res Bull* 1999; 48:319-24.

11. Birdsall, T., et al., "Therapeutic applications of taurine," *Altern Med Rev* 1998; 3:128-36.

12. Kumata, K., et al., "Restoration of endothelium-dependant relaxation in both hypercholesterolemic and diabetics by chronic taurine," *Eur J. Pharmacol* 1996; 303:47-53.

13. Lombardini, J., et al., "Taurine retinal function," *Brain Res Brain Res Rev* 1991; 16(2):151-69.

14. Zackheim, H., et al., "Taurine and psoriasis," *J. Invest Dermatol* 1968; 50(23):277-30.

15. Nakagawa, M., et al., "Antihypertensive effect of taurine on the salt-induced hypertension," *Adv Exp Med Biol* 1994; 359:197-206.

16. Fujita, T., "Hypotensive effect of taurine," Possible involvement of the sympathetic nervous system and endogenous opiates," *J. Clin Invest* 1988; 82(3):993-7.

17. Desai, T., et al., "Taurine deficiency after intensive chemotherapy and/or radiation," *Am J. Clin Nutr* 1992; 55(3):708-11.

18. Paauw., J., et al., "Taurine supplementation at three different dosages and its effect on trauma patients," *Am J. Clin Nutr* 1994; 60(2):203-6.

19. Collins, B., "Plasma and urinary taurine in epilepsy," *Clin Chem* 1988; 34(4):671-5.

Chapter 14

1. Ibid., Klatz, *The New Anti-Aging Revolution*, p. 254.

2. Ibid., Klatz, *The New Anti-Aging Revolution*, p. 255.

3. Ibid., *Great Smokies Interpretative Studies*.

Chapter 15

1. Ibid., Sahley, *Healing with Amino Acids*, p. 50-51.

2. Ibid., Klatz, *The New Anti-Aging Revolution*, p. 256-257.

3. Ibid., *Great Smokies Interpretative Studies*.

Chapter 16

1. Ibid., Sahley, *Healing with Amino Acids*, p. 52.

2. Ibid., Sahley, *Healing with Amino Acids*, p. 49.

3. den Boer, J., et al., "Behavior, neuroendocrine, and biochemical effects of 5-hydroxytryptophan administration in panic disorder," *Psychiatry Res* 1990; 31:267-78.

4. Ribeiro, C., et al., "5-hydroxytryptophan in the prophylaxis of chronic tension-type headache: a double-blind, random, placebo-controlled study for the Portuguese Head Society," *Headache* 2000; 40:451-6.

5. Birdshell, T., "5-hydroxytryptophan: a clinically-effective serotonin precursor," *Alt. Med Rev* 1998; 3:271-8.

Chapter 17

1. Ibid., Klatz, *The New Anti-Aging Revolution*, p. 258.

2. Ibid., Klatz, *The New Anti-Aging Revolution*, p. 259.

3. Ibid., *Great Smokies Interpretative Studies*.

4. Ibid., Klatz, *The New Anti-Aging Revolution*, p. 259.

Section 6

Chapter 1

1. Heller, L., *Applying the Essentials of Herbal Care*. Gig Harbor, Washington: Functional Medicine Institute, 1999.

2. Ibid., Collins, p. 230.

Chapter 2

1. Ibid., Klatz, *The New Anti-Aging Revolution*, p. 272-273.

Chapter 3

1. Moya-Camarena, S., et al., "Conjugated linoleic acid is a potent naturally occurring ligand and activator of PPAR," *J. Lipid Res* 1999; 40:1426-33.

2. Riserus, U., "Conjugated linoleic acid (CLA) reduced abdominal adipose tissue in obese middle-aged men with signs of metabolic syndrome: a randomized controlled trial," *Int J. Obes Relat Metab Disord* 2001; 25(8):1129-35.

3. Blankson, H., et al., "Conjugated linoleic acid reduces body fat mass in overweight and obese humans," *J. Nutr* 2000; 130(12):2943-48.

4. Pariza, M., et. al., "Conjugated dienoic derivatives of linolic acid: a new class of anticarcinogens," *Med Oncol Tumor Pharmacother* 1990; 7(2-3):169-71.

5. Belury, M., et al., "Conjugated dienoic linoleate: a polyunsaturated fatty acid with unique chemorotective properties," *Nur Res* 1995; 53(4Pt 1):83-9.

6. Epstein, F., et al., "Glucose transporters and insulin action: implication for insulin resistance and diabetes mellitus," *NEJM* 1999; 341(4):248-57.

7. Ryder, J., et al., "Isomer-specific antidiabetic properties of conjugated linoleic acid. Improve glucose tolerance, skeletal muscle insulin action, and UCP-2 gene expression," *Diabetes* 2001; 50:1149-57.

8. Doyle, L., et al., "Scientific forum explores CLA knowledge," *Inform* 1998; 9(1):69-72.

Chapter 4

1. Crayhon, R., *The Carnitine Miracle*. New York: M. Evans and Company, Inc., 1998.

2. Ibid., Sahley, *Heal with Amino Acids*, p. 28-31.

3. Ibid., Klatz, *The New Anti-Aging Revolution*, p. 229.

4. Ibid., Bland, *Clinical Nutrition: A Functional Approach*, p. 50-51.

5. Ibid., Bland, *Applying Functional Medicine in Clinical Practice*, p. 16.

6. Tanphaichitr, V., et al., "Carnitine metabolism and carnitine deficiency," *Nur* 1993; 9:246-254.

7. Ibid., Gaby, *Nutritional Therapy in Medical Practice*, p. 50.

8. Ibid., Gaby, *Nutritional Therapy in Medical Practice*, p. 50.

9. Retter, A., et al., "Carnitine and its role in cardiovascular disease," *Heart Disease* 1999; 1:108-113.

10. Arockia, R., et al., "Carnitine as a free radical scavenger in aging," *Exp. Gerontol* 2001; 36:1713-26.

11. De Angelis, C., et al., "Levocarnitine acetyl stimulates peripheral nerve regeneration and neuromuscular junction remodeling following sciatic nerve injury," *In J. Clin Pharmacol Re* 1992; 12:269-79.

12. Ibid., Crayhon, *The Carnitine Miracle*.

13. Brooks, J., et al., "Acetyl-L-Carnitine slows decline in younger patients with Alzheimer's disease: a reanalysis of a double-blind, placebo-controlled study using the trilinear approach," *Int Psychogeriatr* 1998; 10:192-203.

14. Spoganoli, A., et al., "Long-term acetyl-L-carnitine treatment in Alzheimer's disease," *Neurology* 1991; 41:1726-32.

15. Garzya, G., et al., "Evaluation of the effects of L-acetylcarnitine on senile patients suffering from depression," *Drugs Exp. Clin Res* 1990; 16:101-6.

Chapter 5

1. Boldyrev, A., et al., "The antioxidative properties of carnosine, a natural histidine containing dipeptide," *Biochem Int* 1987; 15:1105-13.

2. Hipkiss, A., et al., "Carnosine protects proteins against methylglycoxal-mediated modifications," *Bochem Biophys Res Comm* 1998; 248(1):28-32.

3. Boldyrev, A., "Biochemical and physiological evidence that carnosine is an endogenous neuroprotector against free radicals," *Cell Mol Neurobiol* 1997; 17(2):259-71.

4. Horning, M., et al., "Endogenous mechanisms of neuro-protection: role of zinc, copper, and carnosine," *Brain Res* 2000; 852(1):56-61.

5. Gulyaeva, N., et al., "Superoxide-scavenging activity of carnosine in the presence of copper and zinc ions," *Biochemistry (Masc)* 1987; 52(7 Part 2):1051-54.

6. Wang, A., et al., "Use of carnosine as a natural anti-senescence drug for human beings," *Biochemistry (Masc)* 2000; 65:869-71.

7. Stvolinsky, S., et al., "Anti-ischemic activity of carnosine," *Biochemistry (Masc)* 2000; 65:849-55.

8. Price, D., et al., "Chelating activity of advanced glycation end-product inhibitors," *Jour Bio Chem* 2001; 276:48967-72.

9. Ririe, D., et al., "Vasodilatory actions of the dietary peptide carnosine," *Nutrition* 2000; 16:168-72.

10. Stvolinsky, S., et al., "Carnosine: an endogenous neuroprotector in the ischemic brain," *Cell Mol Neurobiol* 1999; 19:4556.

11. Quinn, P., et al., "Carnosine: its properties, functions, and potential therapeutic applications," *Mol Aspects Med* 1992; 13:379-444.

12. Roberts, OP, et al., "Dietary peptides improve wound healing following surgery," *Nutrition* 1998; 14:266-9.

13. "The anti-aging effects of carnosine," *Life Extensions* 2003; Jan, p. 56-62.

Chapter 6

1. Sinatra, S., *The Coenzyme Q-10 Phenomenon*. New Canaan, CT: Keats Publishing Inc., 1998.

2. Ibid., Sinatra, The Coenzyme Q-10 Phenomenon, p. 29.

3. Perlmutter, D., "The Basic Science of Neurodegenerative Disease," *Brain Biochemistry and Nutrition*. Gig Harbor Washington: Functional Medicine Institute, 2002 p. 159.

4. Mortensen, S., et al., "Dose-related decrease of serum coenzyme Q-10 during treatment with HMG-COA reductase inhibitors," *Mol Aspects of Med* 1997; 18(suppl):S137-44.

5. Ibid., Perlmutter, "The Brain on Fire" p. 179.

6. Rozen, T., et al., "Open trial of coenzyme Q-10 as a migraine preventive," *Cephalalgia* 2002; 22(2):137-41.

7. Sinatra, S., "Cutting Edge Technology in the prevention and treatment of cardiovascular disease: alternative interventions in treating cardiovascular disease" A4M Conference Dec. 2003, p. 101.

8. Langsjoen, P. et al., "Overview of the use of coenzyme Q-10 in cardiovascular disease," *Bio Factors* 1999; 9:273-84.

9. Singh, R., et al., "Coenzyme Q-10 and its role in heart disease," *J. Clin Biochem Nutr* 1999; 26:109-118.

10. Hoffman-Bang, C., et al., "Coenzyme Q-10 as an adjunctive treatment of congestive heart failure," *Am J. Cardiol* 1992; supp 19(3):216 A.

11. Singh, R., et al., "Effect of hydro-soluble coenzyme Q-10 on blood pressures and insulin resistance in hypertensive patients with coronary artery disease," *J. Human Hypertension* 1999; 13(3):203-208.

12. Digiesi, V., et. al., "Effect of coenzyme Q-10 on essential hypertension," *Curr Ther Res* 1990; 47:841-45.

13. Morisco, C., "Effect of coenzyme Q-10 therapy in patients with congestive heart failure: a long-term multicenter, randomized trial," *Clin Investig* 1993; 71:S134-S136.

14. Burke, B., et al., "Randomized double-blind, placebo-controlled trial of coenzyme Q-10 in isolated systolic hypertension," *Southern Med J.* 2001; 94(11):1112-17.

15. Ibid., Sinatra, *Coenzyme Q-10 Phenomenon*.

16. Ibid., Sinatra, "New and Alternative Interventions for Preventing and Treating Cardiovascular Disease," p. 103.

17. Ibid., Sinatra, *Heart Sense for Women*, p. 108.

Chapter 7

1. Rountree, R., *Immunotics*. New York: Berkley Publishing Group, 2000, p. 193.

2. Burke, V., et al., "Dietary protein and soluble fiber reduce ambulatory blood pressure in treatment of hypertensives," *Hypertension* 2001; 38(4):821-26.

3. Ibid., Houston, *What Your Doctor May Not Tell You About Hypertension*, p. 147-48.

4. Ibid., Houston, *What Your Doctor May Not Tell You About Hypertension*, p. 147-48.

Chapter 8

1. Sahley, B. *GABA: The Anxiety Amino Acid*. San Antonio, Texas: Pain & Stress Publications, 1999.

2. Ibid., Klatz, *The New Anti-Aging Revolution*, p. 236.

3. Ibid., Sahley, *GABA: The Anxiety Amino Acid*, p. 16.

4. Ibid., Klatz, *The New Anti-Aging Revolution*, p. 236.

Chapter 9

1. Ibid., Klatz, *The New Anti-Aging Revolution*, p. 289-90.

2. Ibid., Crayhon, *Nutrition Made Simple*, p. 173-81.

3. Sendl, A., et al., "Inhibition of cholesterol synthesis in vitro by extracts and isolated copounds prepared from garlic and wild garlic." *Atherosclerosis* 1992:94:79-86.

4. Jarrell, S., et al., "Effects of wild garlic (allium ursinum) on blood pressure in systolic hypertension," *J. Amer Coll Nur* 1996; 15:532.

5. Ackermann, R., et al., "Garlic shows promise for improving some cardiovascular risk factors," *Arch Inter Med* 2001; 151:813-24.

6. Ibid., Liberman, *The Real Vitamin and Mineral Book*, p. 203-204.

7. Ibid., Rountree, *Immunotics*, p. 99.

8. Pedraza-Chaverri, J., et al., "Garlic prevents hypertension induced by chronic inhibition of nitric oxide synthesis," *Life Sci* 1998; 62:71-77.

9. Orckhov, A., et al., "Effects of garlic on atherosclerosis," *Nutrition* 1997; 13:656-63.

10. McMahon, F., et al., "Can garlic lower blood pressure? A pilot study," *Pharmaccotherapy* 1993; 13:406-407.

11. Silagy, C., et al., "A meta-analysis of the effect of garlic on blood pressure," *J. Hypertens.* 1994; 12:463-68.

Chapter 10

1. Ibid., Packer, *The Antioxidant Miracle*, p. 117-18.

2. LeBars, P., et al., "A placebo-controlled, double-blind, random trial of an extract of ginkgo biloba for dementia," *JAMA* 1997; 278:1327-32.

3. Kleijnen, J., et al., "Ginkgo biloba for cerebral insufficiency," *Br. J. Clin Pharmacol* 1992; 34(4):352-58.

4. Lebars, P., et al., "Ginkgo biloba for dementia," *JAMA* 1997; 278:1327-32.

5. Haramski, N., et al., "Effects of natural antioxidant ginkgo biloba extract (EGB 761) on myocardial ischemia-reperfusion injury," *Free Radic Biol Med* 1994; 16(6):789-94.

6. Akiba, S., et al., "Inhibitory effect of the leaf extract of ginkgo biloba on oxidative stress-induced platelet aggregation," *Biochem Mol Bio. Int* 1998; 46(6):1243-48.

7. Sikora, R., et al., "Ginkgo biloba extract in the therapy of erectile dysfunction," *J Urol* 1989; 141:188A.

8. Chang, H., et al., "Ginkgo biloba extract increases ocular blood flow velocity," *J. Ocul Pharmacol Therapy* 1999; 15(3):233-40.

9. Meyer, B., et al., "A multi-center, double-blind, drug vs. placebo study of gingko biloba extract in the treatment of tinnitus," *Prese Med* 1986; 5:1562-64.

Chapter 11

1. Ibid., Collins, 239-40.

2. Ibid., Klatz, *The New Anti-Aging Revolution*, p. 296.

Chapter 12

1. Ibid., Klatz, *The New Anti-Aging Revolution*, p. 240.

2. Ibid., Klatz, *The New Anti-Aging Revolution*, p. 241.

3. Ibid., Perlmutter, *BrainRecovery.com*, p. 18.

4. Ibid., Klatz, *The New Anti-Aging Revolution*, p. 240.

5. Ibid., Klatz, *The New Anti-Aging Revolution*, p. 240.

Chapter 13

1. Ibid., Klatz, *The New Anti-Aging Revolution*, p. 302.

2. Ibid., Klatz, *The New Anti-Aging Revolution*, p. 302.

Chapter 14

1. J. Nutr 2003; July,133:2470S-2475S.

2. Michnovicz, J., et al., "Induction of estradiol metabolism by dietary indole-3-carbinol in humans," *J. Nat Cancer Inst* 1990; 82:9470-989.

3. Michnovicz, J., et al., "Changes in levels of urinary metabolites after oral indole-3-carbinol in humans," *J. Nat Cancer Inst* 1997; 89(10):718-23.

4. Bradlow, H., et al., "Indole-3-carbinol. A novel approach to breast cancer prvention," Ann NY Acad Sci 1995; 768:180-200.

5. Chinni, S., et al., "Indole-3-carbinol (I3C) induced cell growth inhibition, GI cell cycle arrest and apoptosis in prostate cancer cells," *Oncogene* 20:2927-36.

Chapter 15

1. Ibid., Berkson, p. 12.

2. Ibid., Berkson, p. 14.

3. Ibid., Berkson, p. 101.

4. Packer, L., et al., "Neuroprotection by the metabolic antioxidant alpha lipoic acid," *Free-radical Biology and Medicine* 1997; 22:359-78.

5. Ibid., Packer, *The Antioxidant Miracle*, p. 31.

6. Ibid., Berkson, p. 119.

7. Ibid., Berkson, p. 88.

8. Ibid., Berkson, p. 119.

9. Ibid., Berkson, p. 141.

10. Ibid., Berkson, p. 18.

11. Ibid., Berkson, xv-xvi.

12. Jacob, S., et al., "Enhancement of glucose disposal in patients with type 2 diabetes by alpha lipoic acid.," *Arzneimittel-Forshung/Drug Research* 1995; 45:872-74.

13. Nagamatsu, M., et al., "Lipoic acid improves nerve blood flow, reduces oxidative stress and improves distal nerve conduction in experimental diabetic neuropathy," *Diabetes Care* 1995; 18:1160-67.

14. Packer, L., et al., "Alpha-lipoic acid: a metabolic antioxidant which regulates NF-kappaB signal transduction and protects against oxidative injury," *Drug Metab Rev* 1998; 30(2):245-75.

15. Estrada. D., et al., "Stimulation of glucose uptake by the natural coenzyme alpha-lipoic acid/thiotic acid: participation of elements of the insulin signaling pathway." *Diabetes* 1996; 45(12):1798-804.

Chapter 16

1. Poeggeler, B., et al., "Melatonin—a highly potent endogenous radical scavenger and e-donor: new aspects of the oxidation chemistry of this indole-accessed in vitro," *Ann NY Acad Sci* 1994; 738:419-21.

2. Ibid., Collins, p. 339.

3. Sharkey, K., et al., "Melatonin phase shifts human circadian rhythms in a placebo-controlled simulated night-work study," *Am J. Physiol Regul Integr Comp Physiol* 2002; 282(2):R454-63.

3. Ibid., Collins, p. 339.

4. Ibid., Collins, p. 339.

5. Ibid., Collins, P. 239.

6. Ram, P., et al., "Estrogen receptor transactivation in MCF-7 breast cancer cells by melatonin and growth factors," *Mol Cell Endocrinol* 1998; 141(1-2):53-64.

7. Cos, S., et al., "Influence of melatonin on invasive and metastic properties of MCF-7 human breast cancer cells," *Cancer Res* 1998; 58(19):4383-90.

Chapter 17

1. Leng-Peschlow, E., et al., "Properties and medical use of flavonolignans (silymarin) from silybum marianum," *Phytother Res* 1996; 10(Suppl):S24-S26.

2. Dehmlow, C., et al., "Scavenging of reactive oxygen species and inhibition of arachidonic acid metabolism by silibinin in human cells," *Life Sci* 1996; 58:1591-1600.

3. Skuttowa, M., et al., "Activity of silymarin and its flavonolignans upon low density lipoproteins oxidizability in vitro," *Phytother Res* 1999; 12:535-37.

4. Skottowa, N., et al., "Silymarin as a potential hypocholesterolemic drug," *Physiol Res* 1998; 47:1-7.

5. Dehmlow, C., et al., "Inhibition of Kepffer cell functions as an explanation for the hepatoprotene properties of silibinin," *Hepatology* 1996; 23(4):749-54.

6. Velussi, M., et al., "Long-term treatment with antioxidant drug (silymarin) is effective on hyperinsulinemia, exogenous insulin need and malondialdehyde in cirrhotic diabetic patients," *J. Hepatol* 1997; 26(4):871-79.

7. Bokemeyer, C., et al., "Silibinin protects against cisplatin-induced nephro-toxicity without compromising cisplatin or iposfamide anti-tumor activity," *Br. J. Cancer* 1996; 74:2036-41.

Chapter 18

1. Jacob, S., The Miracle of MSM. New York: Penguin Putnam, 1999, p. 10-11, 23.

2. Ibid., Jacob, p. 3.

3. Ibid., Jacob, p. 32.

Chapter 19

1. Ibid., Klatz, *The New Anti-Aging Revolution*, p. 316.

2. Halpern, M., et al., "Red wine polyphenols an inhibiton of platelet aggregation: possible mechanisms and potential use in heatlh promotions and disease preventions,"*J. Int Med Res* 1998; 26(4):171-180.

3. Ibid., Klatz, *The New Anti-Aging Revolution*, p. 317.

4. Preuss, H., et al., "Effects of niacin bound chromium and grape seed proanthocyanidin extract on the lipid profile of hypercholesterolemic subjects: a pilot study," *J. Med* 2000; 31(5-6):227-46.

5. Noir, N., et al., "Grape seed extract activates Th1 cells in vitro," Clin Diagn Lab Immunol 2002; 9(2):470-76.

6. Ibid., Klatz, *The New Anti-Aging Revolution*, p. 236.

7. Ibid., Sinatra, *Heart Sense for Women*, p. 115.

Chapter 20

1. Kidd., P., et al., "Phosphatidylcholine: a superior protectant against liver damage," *Alt Med Rev* 1996; 1(4):258-74.

2. Olszewsik, A., et al., "Reduction of plasma lipid and homocysteine levels by pyridoxine, folate, cobalamin, choline, riboflavin, and troxerutin in atherosclerosis," *Atherosclerosis* 1989; 5(1):1-6.

3. Little, A., et al., "A double-blind, Placebo controlled trial of high-dose lecithin in Alzheimer's disease. *J. Neurol Neurosurg*, Psychiatry 1985; 4 8(8):736-42.

4. Barbagallo, S., "Alpha-GPC in the mental recovery of cerebral ischemic attacks, an Italian multicenter clinical trial," *Ann NY Acad Sc* 1994; 717:253-269.

Chapter 21

1. Monteleone, P., et al., "Effects of phyosphatidylserine on the neuroendocrine response to physical stress in humans," *Neuroendocrinology* 1990; 52:243-48.

2. Ibid., Schmidt, *Brain-Building Nutrition*, p. 192.

3. Kidd, P., *Phosphatidylserine*. New Canaan, CT: Keats Publishing, Inc., 1998.

4. Ibid., Kidd.

5. Amaducci, L., et al., "Phosphatidylserine in the dosing of Alzheimers disease: results of a multi-center study," *Psychopharmacology Bulletin* 24:130-34.

6. Cenacchi, T., et al., "Cognitive decline in the elderly: a double-blind, placebo-controlled multicenter study on efficacy of phosphatidylserine administration," *Aging: Clinical and Experiment Res* 1993; 5:123-33.

7. Crook, T., et al., "Effects of phosphatidylserine in age-associated memory impairment," *Neurology* 1991; 4:644-49.

8. Crook, T., et al., "Effects of phosphatidylserine in Alzheimer's disease," *Psychopharmacology Bulletin* 1992; 28:61-66.

9. Engel, R., et al., "Double-blind cross-over, study of phosphatidylserine vs. placebo in sugjects with early cognitive deterioration of the Alzheimer's type," *Europen Neuropsychopharmacology* 1992; 2:149-55.

10. Heiss, W., et al., "Long-term effects of phosphatidylserine, pyritinol, and cognitive training in Alzheimer's disease," *Cognitive Deterioration* 1994; 5:88-98.

11. Monteleone, P., et al., "Effects of phosphatidylserine on the neuroendocrine response to physical stress in humans," *Neuroendocrinology* 1990; 52:243-8.

12. Monteleone, P., et al., "Blunting of chronic phosphatidylserine administration of the stress-induced activation of the hypothalamo-pituitary adrenal axis in healthy men," *Eur Jour of Clin Pharm* 1992; 41:385-88.

Chapter 23

1. Ibid., Packer, *The Antioxidant Miracle*, p. 125-27.

Chapter 24

1. Ibid., Heller, *Healthy Women, Healthy Aging*, p. 50.

2. Lu, R., "Resveratrol, a natural product derived from grape, exhibits antiestrogenic activity and inhibits the growth of human breast cancer cells," *J. Cell Physiol* 1999; 179:297-304.

3. Hiroyuki, N., et al., "Resveratrol inhibits human breast cancer cell growth and may mitigate the effect of linoleic acid, a potent breast cancer cell stimulator," *J. Cancer Res Clin Oncol* 2001; 127:258-64.

4. Mitchell, T, "Resveratrol: Cutting-Edge Technology Available Today," *Life Extensions December*, 2003 (Suppl).

5. Zbikowska, H., et al., "Antioxidants with carcinostatic activity (reseveratrol, vitamin E, and selenium) in modulation of platelet adhesion," *J. Physiol Pharmacol* 2000; 51:513-20.

6. Jang, J., et al., "Protective effect of reservatrol on beta-amyloid-induced oxidative PC12 cell death," *Free Radic Biol Med* 2003; 34:1100-10.

7. Chanvitayapongs, , S., et al., "Amelioration of oxidative stress by antioxidants and resveratrol in PC12 cells," *Neuro Report* 1997; 8:1499-502.

8. Cal., C., et al., "Resveratrol and cancer: chemoprevention, apoptosis, and chemoimmuno sensitizing activities," *Curr Med Chem Anti Cancer* Agents 2003; 3:77-93.

9. Mitchell, S., et al., "Resveratrol inhibits the express and function of the androgen receptor in LNcaP prostate cancer cells," *Cancer Res* 1999; 59:5892-5.

Chapter 25

1. Ibid., Klatz, *The New Anti-Aging Revolution*, p. 321.

2. Ibid., Collins, p. 244.

Chapter 26

1. Ley, B., et al., *Boost Your Brain Power with Periwinkle Extract*. Detroit Lakes, MN: BL Publications, 2000, p. 16.

2. Ibid., Ley, p. 22.

3. Taiji, H., et al., "Clinical study of vinpocetine in the treatment of vertigo" *JPN Pharmacol Ter* 1986; 14:577.

4. Miyazaki, M., et al., "The effect of a cerebral vasodilator vinpocetine, on cerebral vascular resistance evaluated by the Doppler ultrasonic technique in patients with cerebrovascular diseases," *Angiology* 1995; 46(1):53-8.

Chapter 27

1. Wise, J., et al., "Changes in plasma carotenoid, alpha-tocopherol, and lipid peroxide levels in response to supplementation with concentrated fruit and vegetable extracts: a pilot," *Curr Ther Res* 1996, 57(6):445.

2. Watson, R., et al., "Immune function improves during fruit and vegetable extract supplementation." *Integrative Med* 1999, 2(1):3.

3. Smith, M., et al., "Supplementation with fruit and vegetable extracts reduces DNA damage in the peripheral lymphocytes of an elderly population: a pilot," Nutr Res 1999; 19(10):1507.

Section 7

Chapter 1

1. Crayhon, R., *Designs For Health Institute's Eating and Supplement Plans*. Boulder, CO: Designs for Health Institute, 2000.

2. Sahley, B. *Is Ritalin Necessary?* San Antonio Texas: Pain and Stress Publications, 1999, p. 12.

3. Ibid., Sahley, *Is Ritalin Necessary?* p. 12.

4. Breggin, P., *Talking Back to Ritalin*. Monroe, Maine: Common Conrage Press, 1998.

5. Stevens, L., et al., "Essential fatty acids metabolism in boys with attention-deficit hyperactivity disorder ," *Am J. Clin Nutr* 1995; 62:761-768.

6. Kozielec, T., et al., "Assessment of magnesium levels in children with ADHD," *Magnes Res* 1997; 10:143-48.

7. Starobrat-Hermelin, B., et al., "The effects of magnesium physiological supplementation on hyperactivity in children with ADHD. Positive response to magnesium oral loading test," *Magnes Res* 1997; 10:149-56.

8. Bekaroglu, M., et al., "Relationships between serum free fatty acids and zinc, and ADHD: A research note," *J. Child Psychol Psychiatry* 1996; 37:225-27.

9. Brenner, A., et al., "The effects of megadoses of selected B complex vitamins on children with hyperkinesis: controlled studies with long term followup," *J. Learning Dis* 1982; 15:258.

10. Colquhoun, V., et al., "A lack of essential fatty acids as a possible cause of hyperactivity in children," *Med Hypotheses* 1981; 7:681.

11. Ibid., Sahley, *Control Hyperactivity/ADD Naturally.*

12. Stordy, B., *The LCP Solution.* New York: Balantine Books, 2000, p. 2.

13. Lyon, M., *Healing the Hyperactive Brain.* Calgary AB: Focused Publishing, 2000.

14. Ibid., Crayhon, *Eating and Supplement Plans.*

15. Van Oudheusden, L., et al., "Efficacy of carnitine in the treatment of children with attention-deficit hyperactivity disorder," *Prostaglandins Leukot Essent Fatty Acids* 2002; 67(1):33.

Chapter 2

1. Sahley, B., *Anxiety Epidemic.* San Antonio Texas: Pain & Stress Publications, 1999, p. 65.

2. Sahley, B., *Control Hyperactivity/ADD Naturally*, p. 31.

3. Crayhon, R., *Designs for Health Institute's Level II Eating and Supplement Plans.* Boulder CO: Designs for Health Institute, Inc., 1999.

4. Sult, T., et al., Th1/Th2 balances: a natural therapeutic approach to Th2 polarization in allergy," *Applied Nutritional Science Reports*, 2003; p. 8.

5. Jakazawa, T., et al., "Metabolites of orally administered perilla frutescens extract in rats and humans," *Biol Pharm Bul* 2000; 23(1):122-27.

6. Tate, G., et al., "Suppresion of acute and cronic inflammation by dietary gamma linolenic acid," *J. Rheumatol* 1989; 16(6):729-34.

7. Musonda, C., et al., "Quercetin inhibits hydrogen peroxide (H202)-induced NF-KappaB DNA binding activity and DNA damage in Hep G2 cells," *Carcinogensis* 1998; 19(9):1583-9.

8. Kodama, M., et al., "Autoimmune disease and allergy are controlled by vitamin C treatment," *In Vivio* 1994; 8(2):251-7.

9. Packer, L., et al., "Alpha-lipoic acid as a biological antioxidant," *Free Rad Biol Med* 1995; 19(2):227-50.

10. Chan, M., et al., "Effects of three dietary phytochemicals from tea, rosemary and turmeric on inflammation-induced nitrite production," *Cancer Lett* 1995; 96(1)23-9.

Chapter 3

1. Newman, P., et al., "Could diet be used to reduce the risk of developing Alzheimer's disease?" *Med Hypothesis* 1998; 50:335-37.

2. LeBars, P., et al., "A placebo-controlled double-blind randomized trial of an extract of ginkgo biloba for dementia," *JAMA* 1997; 2789(6):1327-32.

3. Sano, M., et al., "A controlled trial of selegeline, alpha-tocopherol, or both as treatment for Alzheimer's disease," *NEJM* 1997; 336:1216-22.

4. Birkmayer, J., et al., "Coenzyme nicotinamide adenine dinucleotide: new therapeutic approach for improving dementia of the Alzheimer type," *Ann Clin & Lab Sci* 1996; 26(1):1-9.

5. Nourhashemi, F, et al., "Alzheimer's disease: protective factors," *Am J. Clin Nutr* 2000; 71(Suppl):643S-649S.

6. Aisen., P., et al., "Inflammatory mechanisms in Alzheimer's disease: implications for therapy," *Am J. Psychiatr* 1995: 151:1105-13.

7. Christen, Y., et al., "Oxidative stress and Alzheimer's disease," *Am J. Clin Nutr* 2000; 71 (Suppl):621S-629S.

8. Wang., H., et al., "Vitamin B12 and folate in relation to the development of Alzheimer's disease," *Neurology* 1991; 56:1188-94.

9. Pettegrew, J., et al., "Clinical and neuro-chemical effects of acetyl-L-carnitine in Alzheimer's disease," *Neurobiol Aging* 1995; 16(1):1-4.

10. Nichols, T., et al., "Alpha-lipoic acid: biological effects and clinical implications," *Alt Med Rev* 1997; 2(3):177-83.

11. Gottfries, C., et al., "Therapy options in Alzheimer's disease," *BJCP* 1994; 48(6):327-30.

12. Breitner, J., et al., "Inflammatory processes and anti-inflammatory drugs in Alzheimer's disease: a current appraisal," *Neurobiol Aging* 1996; 17(5):789-94.

13. Salvioli, g., et al., "L-acetylcarnitine treatment of mental decline in the elderly," *Drugs Exp Clin Res* 1994; 20:169-76.

14. Villardita, C., et al., "Multicenter clinical trial of brain phosphatidyl serine in elderly patients with intellectual deterioration," *Clin Trials J.* 1987; 24:84-93.

15. Clarke, R., et al., "Folate, vitamin B12, and serum total homocysteine levels in confirmed Alzheimer's disease," *Arch Neurol* 1998; 55:1449-55.

16. Nourhashemi, F., et al., "Alzheimer's disease: protective factors," *Am J. Clin Nutr* 2000; 71(2):643S-649S.

17. Crook, T., et al., "Effects of phosphatidylserine in aged-associated memory impairment," *Neurology* 1991; 41(5):644-649.

18. Thal, L., et al., "A one-year multicenter placebo-controled study of acetyl-L-carnitine in patients with Alzheimer's disease," *Neurology* 1996; 4793):705-11.

19. Laszy, J., et al., "Comparison of cognitive enhancer activity of acetylcho-linesterase inhibitors and vinopcetine," *Neurobiol of Aging* 2002; 23(1)Suppl 1:357.

20. Seshadri, S., "Plasma homocystine as a risk factor for dementia and Alzheimer's disease," *NEJM* 2002; 346:476-83.

21. Conquer, J., et al., "Fatty acid analysis of blood plasma of patients with Alzheimer's disease, other types of dementia, and cognitive impairment," *Lipids* 2000; 35:1305-12.

22. Kyle, D., et al., "Low serum docosahexaenoic acid is a significant risk factor for Alzheimer's dementia," *Lipids* 1999; 34:S245.

23. Kalmijn, S., et al., "Fatty acid intake and the risk of dementia and cognitive decline: a review of clinical and epidemiological studies," *J. Nutr Health Aging* 2000; 4(4):202-07.

24. Sehardi, S., et al., "Plasma homocystine as a risk factor for dementia and Alzheimer's disease," *NEJM* 2002; 346(7):476-83.

25. Nouihashemi, F., et al., "Alzheimer's disease: proactive factors," *Am J. Clin Nutr* 2000; 71(2):643S-49S.

26. Morris, M., et al., "Homocysteine and Alzheimer's disease," *Lancet Neurol* 2003; 2(7):425-28.

27. Tenissen, C., et al., "Homocysteine: a marker for cognitive performance? A longitudinal follow-up study," *J. Nutr Health Aging* 2003; 7(3):153-9.

Chapter 4

1. Ward, N., et al., "Assessment of zinc status and oral supplementation in anorexia nervosa," *J. Nutr Med* 1990; 1:171-77.

Chapter 5

1. Ibid., Sahley, *The Anxiety Epidemic*, p. 35.

2. Ibid., Sahley, *The Anxiety Epidemic*, p. 54.

3. Ibid., Gaby, *Nutritional Therapy in Medical Practice*, p. 98-99.

Chapter 6

1. Rountree, R., "Immune Dysfunction and Inflammation, Part II," *Applying Functional Medicine In Clinical Practice*. Gig Harbor, WA: The Institute for Functional Medicine, 2002, p. 1-30.

2. Ibid., Rountree, p. 21.

3. Ibid., Rountree, p. 21.

4. Ibid., Rountree, p. 24.

5. Ibid., Rountree, p. 25.

6. McAlinton, T., et al., "Glucosamine and chondrotin for the treatment of ostoarthritis," *JAMA* 2002; 283:1469-75.

7. Reginster, J., et al., "Long-term effects of glucosamine sulfate on osteoarthritis progress, placebo-controlled trial," *Lancet* 2001; 357:251-56.

8. Srivastava, L., et al., "Ginger (Zingiber officinale) in rheumatism and musculoskeletal disorders," *Med Hypothesis* 1992; 39(4):342-48.

9. Flynn, D., et al., "Inhibition of human neutrophil-lipoxygenase activity by ginger dione shagaol, capsaicin, and related pungent compounds," *Prostaglandins Leukotr Med* 1986; 24:195-98.

10. Sato, M., et al., "Quercetin, a bioflavonoid, inhibits the induction of interleukin gamma and monocyte chemoattractant protein-expression by

tumor necrosis factor-alpha in cultured human synovial cells," *J. Rheumatol* 1997; 24(9):1680-94.

11. Morreale, P., et al., "Comparison of the antiinflamatory efficacy of chondroitin sulfate and dicolfenac sodium in patients with knee osteoarthritis," *J. Rheumatol* 1996; 23:1385-91.

12. Uebelhart, D., et al., "Effects of oral chondrotin sulfate on the progression of knee osteoarthritis: a pilot study," *Osteoarthritis Cartilage* 1998; 6(Suppl A): 39-46.

13. Travers, R., et al., "Boron and arthritis: the results of a double-blind pilot study" *J. Nutr Med* 1990; 1:127-32.

14. Vaz, A., et al., "Double-blind-clinical evaluation of the relative efficacy of ibuprofen and glucosamine sulfate in the management of the knee in out-patients," *Curr Med Resp Opin* 1982; 8:145-49.

15. Drovanti, A., et al., "Therapeutic activity of oral glucosamine sulfate in osteoarthritis: a placebo-controlled, double-blind invetigation," *Clin Ther* 1980; 3:260-72.

16. Di Silvestro, R., et al., "Effects of copper supplementation on ceruloplasmin and copper-zinc superoxide dismutase in free-living rheumatoid arthritis patients," *Amer Jour Clin Nutr* 1992; 11(2):177-80.

17. Zurier, R., et al., "Gamma-linolenic acid treatment of rheumatoid arthritis: a randomized, placebo-controlled trial," *Arthritis Rheum* 1996; 39:1808-17.

18. Leventhal, L., et al., "Treatment of rheumatoid arthritis with black currant seed oil," *Br J. Rheumatol* 1994; 33:847-852.

19. Brzeski, M., et al., "Evening primrose oil in patients with rheumatoid arthritis and side-effects of non-steroidal anti-inflammatory drugs," Br J. Rheumatol 1991; 30:370-72.

20. Kremer, J., et al., "Effects of high-dose fish oil on rheumatoid arthritis after stopping NSAID. Clinical and immune correlates," *Arthritis Rheum* 1995; 38:1107-14.

21. Tarp, U., et al., "Low selenium level in rheumatoid arthritis," *Scan J. Rheumatol* 1985; 14:97-101.

22. Deretz, A., et al., "Adjuvant tretment of recent onset of rheumatoid arthritis by selenium supplementation: preliminary observations," *Br J. Rheumatol* 1992; 31:281-86.

23. Bland, J., "GALT: activation, inflammation, and premature aging," *Improving Genetic Expression in the Prevention of the Diseases of Aging*. Gig Harbor, WA: HealthComm International, Inc., 1998, p. 166-172.

24. Shen, F., et al., "Inhibition of xanthine oxidase by purpurogallin and silymarin group," *Anticancer Res* 1998; 18(1A):263-7.

Chapter 7

1. Ibid., Crayhon, *Eating and Supplement Plans.*

2. Greene, L., et al., "Asthma and oxidant stress: nutritional, environmental, and genetic risk factors," *J. Am Coll Nutr* 1995; 14(4):317-24.

3. ~~Weiss, S., et al., "Diet as a risk factor for asthma," *Ciba Found Symp* 1997;~~ 206:244-57.

4. Hatch, G., et al., "Asthma, inhaled oxidants, and dietary antioxidants," *Am J. Clin Nutr* 1995; 61(3 Suppl):625S-630S.

5. Britton, J., et al., "Dietary magnesium, lung function, wheezing, and airway hyperactivity in a random adult population sample," *Lancet* 1994; 344(8919):357-62.

6. Kadrabova, J., et al., "Selenium status is decreased in patients with intrinsic asthma," *Biol Trac Elem Res* 1996; 52(3):241-48.

7. Villani, F., et al., "Effect of dietary supplementaiton with polyunsaturated fatty acids on bronchial hyperreactivity in subjects with seasonal asthma," *Respiration* 1998; 65(4):265-59.

Chapter 8

1. Ibid., Heller, *Applying the Essentials of Herbal Care*, p. 15.

2. Ibid., Crayhon, *Eating and Supplement Plans.*

3. Calder, P. et al. "N-3 polyunsturated fatty acids and cytokine production in health and disease," *Ann Nutr Metab* 1997; 41(4):203-34.

4. Fernandes, G., et al., "Dietary lipids and risk of autoimmune disease," *Clin Immunopathol* 1994; 7292):193-97.

5. Robinson, D., et al., "Suppression of autoimmune disease by dietary n-3 fatty acids," *J. Lipd Res* 1993; 34(8):1435-44.

6. Ibid., Crayhon, *Level II Eating and Supplement Plans.*

7. Herrick, A., et al., "Dietary intake of micronutrient antioxidants in relation to blood levels in patients with systemic sclerosis," *J. Rheumatol* 1996; 23(4):650-3.

8. Famularo, G., et al., "Carnitine deficiency in scleroderma," (letter) *Immunol Today* 1999; 20(5):246.

Chapter 9

1. Ames, B., et al., "Are vitamins and mineral deficiencies a major cancer risk?' *Nat Rev Center* 2002; 2:694.

2. Ibid., Crayhon, *Eating and Supplement Plans.*

3. Giovannucci, E., et al., "Intake of carotenoids and retinal in relation to risk of prostate cancer," *J. Natl Cancer Instit* 1995; 87:1767-76.

4. Ibid., Colgan, p. 120-24.

5. Xing., N., et al., "Quercein inhibits the expression and function of the androgen receptor in LCCaP prostate cancer cells," *Carcinogenesis* 2002; 22(3):409-14.

6. Heinonen, O., et al., "Prostate cancer and supplementation with alpha-tocophenols and beta-carotene: incidence and mortality in a controlled trial," *J. Natl Cancer Inst* 1998; 90(6):4400-446.

7. Prasad, K., et al., "Vitamin E and cancer prevention: recent advances and future potentials," *J. Amer Coll Nutr* 1992; 11:487-500.

8. Olson, D., et al., "Vitamin A & E; further clues for prostate cancer prevention," *J. Natl Cancer Inst* 1998; 90(6):414-15.

9. Kucuk, O., "Phase II randomized clinical trial of lycopene supplementation before radical prostatectomy," *Cancer Epidemiol Biomarkers Prev* 2001; 10(8):861-68.

10. Clark, L., et al., "Effects of selenium supplementation for cancer prevention in patients with carcinoma of the skin," *JAMA* 1996; 276(24):1957-63.

11. Giovanucci, E., et al., "Folate, methionine, and alcohol intake and risk of colorectal adenoma," *J. Natl Cancer Inst*; 1993; 85:875-84.

12. Mason, J., et al., "Folate and colonic carcinogenesis: searching for a mechanistic understanding," *J. Nutr Biochem* 1994; 5:170-75.

13. Clark, L., et al., "Decreased incidence of prostate cancer with selenium supplementation: results of a double-blind cancer prevention trial," *Br. J. Urol* 1998; 81:730-34.

14. Bradlow, H., et al. "Multifunctional aspects of the action of vitamin C as an antitumor agent," *Ann NY Acad Sci* 1999; 869:204-13.

15. Wong, G., et al., "Dose-ranging study of indole-3-C for breast cancer prevention," *J. Cell Biochem* 1997; 28-29:111-6.

16. Willett, W., et al., "Nutrition and cancer: summary of the evidence," *Cancer Causes and Control* 1996; 7:178-180.

17. White, E., et al., "Relationship between vitamin and calcium supplement use and colon cancer," Cancer Epidemiol Biomarkers Prev 1997; 6:769-74.

18. Giovannucci, E., et. Al., "MVI use, folate and colon cancer in women," *Ann Int Med* 1998; 129:517-24.

19. Overad, K., "Coenzyme Q-10 in health and disease," *European J. of Clin Nutr* 1999; 53(10):764-70.

20. Cram, E., et al., "Indole-3-carbinol inhibits CDK6 expression in human MCF-7 breast cancer cells by disruption 5p1 transcription factor interactions with a composite element in the CDK6 gener promotor," *J. Biol Chem* 2001; 22:276(25):2332-34.

Chapter 10

1. Ibid., Schmidt, *Tired of Being Tired*, p. 148-49.

2. Ibid., Schmidt, *Tired of Being Tired*, p. 149.

3. Ibid., Crayhon, *Eating and Supplement Plans*.

Chapter 11

1. Ibid., Crayhon, *Eating and Supplement Plans*.

2. Nuttall, S, et al., "Antioxidant therapy for the prevention of cardiovascular disease," *Q. J. Med* 1999; 92:239-44.

3. Langsjoen, P., et al., "Overview of the use of coenzyme Q-10 in cardiovascular disease," Bio Factors 1999; 9:273-84.

4. Stampfer, M., et al., "Vitmain E consumption and the risk of cornary disease in women," *NEJM* 1997; 328:144-49.

5. Rinnium, E., et al., "Vitamin E consumption and the risk of coronary disease in men," *NEJM* 1993; 328:1450-56.

6. Plotnick, G., et al., "Effect of antioxidant vitamins on the transient impairment of endothelium-dependent brachial artery vasoactivity following a single high-fat meal," *JAMA* 1997; 276(20):1682-86.

7. Reaven, P., et al., "Effect of dietary antioxidant combinations in humans," *Arterioscler Throm* 1993; 13:590-600.

8. Simon, J., et al., "Vitamin C and cardiovascular disease: a review," *J. Am Coll Nutr* 1992; 11:107-25.

9. Price, J., et al., "Antioxidant vitamins in the prevention of cardiovascular disease," *Eur Heart Jour* 1997; 18:719-27.

1.1

1. Ibid., Colgan, p. 128.

2. Ibid., Braverman, *Hypertension and Nutrition*, p. 128-29.

3. Ibid., Braverman, p. 129.

4. Ibid., Braverman, p. 129.

5. Castano, G., et al., "A long-term study of policosanol in the treatment of intermittent claudication," *Angiology* 2001; 52:115-25.

6. Crespo, E., et al., "Compariative study of the efficacy and tolerability of policosanol and lovastatin in patients with hypercholesterolemia and noninsulin-dependnt diabetes mellitus," *Int Jour Clin Pharm Res* 1999; 19:117-27.

7. Castano, G., et al., "Effects of policosanol and pravastatin in lipid profile, platelet aggregation and endothelemia in older hypercholesterolemic patients," *Int J. Clin Pharm Res* 1999; 19:105-116.

8. Castano, G., et al., "Effects of policosanol on older patients with hypertension and type II hypercholesterolemia," *Drugs in R&D* 2002; 3(3):402-8.

9. Arruzazabala, M., et al., "Comparative study of policosanol, aspirin, and the combination therapy of policosanol-aspirin on platelet aggregation in healthy volunteers," *Pharmacological Res* 1997; 36(4):293-7.

10. Ortensi E., et al., "A comparative study of policosanol versus simvastatin in elderly patients with hypercholesterolemia," *Curr Ther Res* 1997; 58:390-401.

11. Menendez, R., et al., "Policosanol modulates HMG-Co-A reducatase activity in cultured fibroblasts," *Archieves Med Res* 2001; 32:8-12.

12. Mas, R., et al., "Effects of policosanol in patients with type II hypercholesterolemia and additional coronary risk factors," *Clin Pharmacol Ther* 1999; 65:439-47.

13. Alcocer, L., et al., "A comparative study of policosanol versus acipimox in patients with type II hypercholesterolemia," *Int J. Tissue React* 1999; XX(3):85-92.

14. Castans, G., et al., "Effects of policosanol treatment on the susceptibility of low density lipoprotein (LDL) isolated from healthy volunteers to oxidative modification in vitro," *Br J. Clin Pharmacol* 2000; 50(3):255-262.

15. Castano, G., et al., "Effects of policosanol on postmenopausal women with type II hypercholesterolemia," *Gynecol Endocrinol* 2000; 14(3):187-195.

16. Castano, G., et al., "Comparisons of the efficacy and tolerability of policosanol with atorvastatin in elderly patients with type II hypercholesterolemia," *Drugs Ageing* 2003; 20(2):153-63.

17. Satyavati, G., ete al., "Guggulipid: A promising hypolipidemic agent from gum guggul (Commiphora)," *Econ Med Plant Res* 1991; 5:47-80.

18. Singh, R., et al., "Hypolipidemic and antioxidant effects of Commiphora mukul as an adjunct to dietary therapy in patients with hypercholesterolemia," *Cardiovas Drugs Ther* 1994; 8(4):659-64.

19. Singh, K., et al., "Guggulsterone, a potent hypolipidaemic, prevents oxidation of low density lipoprotein," *Phytother Res* 1997; 11:291-94.

20. Verma, S., et al., "Effect of Commiphora mukul (gum guggulu) in patients with hyperlipidemia with special reference to HDL cholesterol," *Indian J. Med Res* 1988; 87:356-60.

21. Nityanand, S., et al., "Clinical trials with guggulipid—a new hypolipidaemic agent from gum gugul," *Econ Med Plant Res* 1991; 5:47-82.

22. Tomeo, A., et al., "Antioxidant effects of tocotrienols in patients with hyperlipidemia and carotid stenosis," Lipids 1995; 12:1179-83.

23. Qureshi, A., et al., "Novel tocotrienols of rice bran modulate cardiovascular disease risk paramteters of hypercholesterolemic humans," *Nutritional Biochem* 1997; 8:290-98.

24. Adler, A., et al., "Effect of garlic and fish oil supplementation on serum lipid and lipoprotein concentration in hypercholesterolemic men," *Ann J. Clin Nutr* 1997; 65:445-50.

25. Warshafsky, E., et al., "Effect of garlic on total serum cholesterol," *Ann Int Med* 1993; 119:599-605.

26. Ibid., Crayhon, "Aging Well in the 21st Century," p. 22.

27. Galeone, F., et al., "The lipid-lowering effect of panthethine in hyperlipidemic patients: a clinical investigation," *Curr Ther Res* 1983; 34:383.

28. Maggi, G., et al., "Pantethine: a physiological lipomodulating agent, in the treatment of hyperlipidemias," *Curr Ther Res* 1982; 32:380.

29. Avogaro, P., et al., "Effect of pantethine on lipids, lipoproteins and apolipoproteins in man," *Curr Ther Res* 1983; 33:488.

30. Ibid., Gaby, *Nutritional Therapy in Medical Practice*, p. 47.

31. Gaddi, A., et al., "Controlled evaluation of pantethine, a natural ~~hyplipidemic compound, in patients with different forms of~~ hyperlipoproteinemia," *Atherosclerosis* 1984; 50:73.

32. Maioli, M., et al., "Effect of pantethine on the subfractions of HDL in dyslipemic patients," *Curr Ther Res* 1984; 35:307.

33. Head, K., et al., "Inositol hexaniacinate a safer alternative to niacin," *Alt Med Rev* 1996; 1(3):176-84.

34. Heber, D., et al., "Cholesterol-lowering effects of a proprietary Chinese red-yeast-rice dietary supplement," *Am J. Clin Nutr* 1999; 69:231-36.

35. Anderson, J. et al., "High-fiber diets for diabetic and hypertriglyceridemic patients," *Can Med Assoc J.* 1980; 123:975.

36. Anderson, J., et al., "Oat-bran cereal lowers serum total and LDL cholesterol in hypercholesterolemic men," *Am J. Clin Nutr* 1990; 52:495-99.

37. Wolever, T., et al., "Psyllium reduces blood lipids in men and women with hyperlipidemia," *Am J. Med Sci* 1994; 307:269-73.

38. Sprecher, D., et al., "Efficacy of psyllium in reducing serum cholesterol levels in hypercholesterolemic patients on high-or low-fat diets," *Ann Int Med* 1993; 119:545-54.

39. Ornish, D., et al., "Can lifestyle changes reverse coronary heart disease? *Lancet* 1990; 336:129-33.

40. Press, R., et al., "The effect of chromium picolinate on serum cholesterol and apolipoprotein fractions in human subjects," *West J. Med* 1990; 152:41-45.

41. Urberg, M., et al., "Hypocholesterolemic effects of nicotinic acid and chromium supplementation," *J. Family Pract* 1988; 27:603-06.

42. Davis, W., et al., "Monotherapy with magnesium increases abnormally low high density lipoprotein cholesterol: a clinical assay," *Curr Ther Res* 1984; 36:341-46.

43. Pola, P. et al., "Statistical evaluation of long-term L-carnitine therapy in hyperlipoproteinaemias," *Drugs Expti Clin Res* 1983; 9:925-34.

1.2

1. Gittleman, A., *Super Nutrition for Menopause.* New York: Avery Publishing Group, 1998, p. 87.

2. Maebashi, M. et al., "Lipid-lowering effect of carnitine in patients with type IV hyperlipoproteinemia," *Lancet* 1978; 805-08.

3. Jain, S., et al., "Effect of modest vitamin E supplementation on blood glycated hemoglobin and triglyceride levels and red cell indices in Type I diabetic patients," *J. Am Coll Nutr* 1996; 15(5):458-61.

4. Ibid., Crayhon, "Aging Well in the 21st Century," p. 22.

5. Ibid., Crayhon, "Aging Well in the 21st Century," p. 27.

1.3

1. McCully, K., "Homocysteine and the heart revolution," *Disorders of Intercellular Mediators and Messengers, Their Relationship to Funcitonal Illness.* Gig Harbor, WA: The Functional Medicine Institute, 1999; p. 87.

2. Ibid., Sinatra, *Heart Sense for Women*, p. 53-54.

3. Ford, E., et al., "Homocysteine and cardiovascular disease: a systemic review of the evidence with special emphasis on case-control studies and nested case-control studies," *Int J. Epidemiol* 2002; 31(1):59-70.

4. Clarke, R., et al., "Underestimation of the importance of homocysteine as a risk factor for cardiovascular disease in epidemiological studies," *J. Cardiovasc Risk* 2001; 8(6):363-9.

5. Ibid., Sinatra, *Heart Sense for Women*, p. 55.

6. Ibid., Sinatra, *Heart Sense for Women*, p. 55.

7. Ibid., McCully, "Homocysteine and the heart revolution," p. 87.

8. Talova, J., et al., "Changes of plasma total homocysteine levels during the menstrual cycle," *Eur J. Clin Invest* 1999; 29(12):1041-44.

9. Stoney, C., et al., "Plasma homocysteine levels increase in women during psychological stress," *Life Sci* 1999; 64(25):2359-65.

10. DeCree, C., et al., "Influence of exercise and menstrual cycle phase on plasma homocysteine levels in young women—prospective study," *Scand J. Med Sci Sports* 1999; 9(5):272-78.

11. Bland, J., "Introduction to neuroendocrine disorders," *Functional Medicine Approaches to Endocrine Disturbances of Aging.* Gig Harbor, WA: The Functional Medicine Institute, 2001; p. 61.

12. McCully, D., et al., "Homocystine and vascular disease," *Natur Med* 1996; 2:386-389.

13. Clarke, R., et al., "Hyperhomocysteinemia: an independent risk factor for vascular disease," *NEJM* 1991; 324:1149-55.

14. Glueck, C., et al., "Evidence that homocysteine is an independent risk factor for atherosclerosis in hyperlipidemic patients," *Am J. Cardiol* 1995; 75:132-36.

15. Hackam, D., et al., "What level of homocysteine should be treated? Effects of vitamin therapy on progression of carotid atherosclerosis in patients with homocysteine levels of above and below 14 micromol," *Am J. Hypertens* 2000; 13:105-110.

16. Nygard, O., et al., "Plasma homocysteine levels and mortality in patients with coronary artery disease," *NEJM* 1997; 337:230-36.

17. Petersen, J., et al., "Vitamins and progression of atherosclerosis in hyperhomocysteinemia," *Lancet* 1998; 351:263.

18. McCully, K., et al., "Homocysteine, folate, vitamin B6 and cardiovascular disease," *JAMA* 1998; 279:392-93.

19. Rimm, E., et al., "Folate and vitamin B6 from diet and supplements in relation to risk of coronary artery disease among women," *JAMA* 1998; 279:359-64.

20. Houston, M., "Case Studies in Hypertension: Dietary and Nutraceutical Interventions," *The Heart on Fire: Modifiable Factors Beyond Cholesterol, Workshop.* Gig Harbor, WA: The Institute for Functional Medicine, 2003, p. 129-31.

21. Ibid., Sinatra, *Heart Sense for Women*, p. 53.

22. Ibid., McCully, "Homocysteine and the Heart Revolution," p. 87.

23. Molloy, A., et al., "Thermolabile variant of 5, 10-methylenetetrahydrofolate reductase associated with low red-cell folates: implications for folate intake recommendations," *Lancet* 1997; 249:1591-93.

24. Fodinger, M., et al., "Molecular biology of 5,10-methylenetetrahydrofolate reductase," *J. Nephrol* 1999; 13(1); 20-33.

1.4

1. Ibid., Sinatra, *Heart Sense for Women*, p. 62.

1.5

1. Ibid., Sinatra, *Heart Sense for Women*, p. 63.

2. Matsumoto, Y., et al., "High level of lipoprotein (a) is a strong predictor for progression of coronary artery disease," *J. Atheroscler Throm* 1998; 5(2):47-53.

3. Ridker, P., et al., "Novel risk factors for systemic atherosclerosis: a comparison of C-reactive protein, fibrinogen, homocysteine, lipoprotein (a) and standard cholesterol screening as predictors of peripheral arterial disase," *JAMA* 2001; 285(19):2481-85.

4. Ibid., Sinatra, *Heart Sense for Women*, p. 63.

5. Ibid., Siantra, *Heart Sense for Women*, p. 64.

6. Ibid., Houston, "Case Studies in Hypertension: Dietary and Nutraceutical Interventions," p. 129-31.

7. Sinatra, S., "Preventive Cardiology II," *Longevity and Preventive Medicine Symposium.* 2002, p. 9.

1.6

1. Ibid., Sinatra, *Heart Sense for Women*, p. 66.

2. Rost, N., et al., "Plasma concentration of C-reactive protein and risk of ischemic stroke and transient ischemic attack: the Framingham study," *Stroke* 2001; 32(11):2575-79.

3. Ibid., Ridker, p. 2481-85.

4. Jialal, I., "Inflammation and atherosclerosis: the value of the high-sensitivity c-reactive protein assay as a risk marker," *Am J. Clin Pathol* 2001; 116, Suppl:S108-15.

5. Teunissen, C., et al., "Inflammation markers in relation to cognition in a healthy aging population," *J. Neuroimmunol* 2003; 134(1-2):142-50.

6. Miller, G., et al., "Clinical depression and inflammatory risk markers for coronary artery disease," *Am J. Cardiol* 2002; 90(12):1279-83.

7. Pradhan, A., et al., "Do atherosclerosis and type 2 diabetes share a common inflammatory basis? *Eur Heart Jour* 2002; 23(11):831-4.

8. Ibid., Sinatra, *Heart Sense for Women*, p. 66.

9. Madsen, T., et al., "C-reactive protein, dietary n-3 fatty acids, and the extent of coronary artery disease," *Am J. Cardiol* 2001; 88(10):1139-42.

10. Ford, E., et al., "Does exercise reduce inflammation? Physical activity and c-reactive protein among U.S. adults," *Epidemiology* 2002; 13(5):561-8.

11. Ridker, P., et al., "C-reactive protein and other markers of inflammation in the prediction of cardiovascular disease in women," *NEJM* 2000; 342:836-43.

12. Devara, S.,et al., "Alpha tocopherol supplementation decreases serum c-reactive protein and monocyte interleukin-6 levels in normal volunteers and type 2 diabetic patients," *Free Radical Biol Med* 2000; 29(8):790-92.

13. Rifai, N., et al., "Inflammatory markers and coronary artery disease," *Curr Opin Lipidol* 2002; 4:383-89.

14. Albert, C., et al., "Prospective study of c-reactive protein, homocysteine, and plasma lipid levels as predictors of sudden cardiac death," *Circulation* 2002; 105(22):2595-99.

15. Rifai, N., et al., "C-reactive protein and coronary heart disease," *Cardiovasc Toxicol* 2001; 1(2):153-57.

1.7

1. Ibid., Crayhon, "Aging Well in the 21st Century," p. 22.

Chapter 12

1. Crayhon, R., "Nutritional Medicine Update," Seminar 2003, p. 32.

Chapter 14

1. Ibid., Gaby, *Nutritional Therapy in Medical Practice*, p. 68.

2. Dzugan, S., "Natural Approaches in the treatment of congestive heart failure" *Life Extension* 2003; Dec. p. 61-68.

3. Morelli, V., et al., "Alternative therapies: part II, congestive heart failure and hypercholesterolemia," *Am Fam Physician* 2000; 62(6):1325-30.

4. Gavagan, T., et al., "Cardiovascular disease," *Prim Care* 2002; 29(2):323-38.

5. Sole, M., et al., "Conditioned nutritional requirements and the pathogenesis and treatment of myocardial failure," *Curr Opin Clin Nutr Metabolic Care* 2000; 3(6):417-24.

6. Morisco, C., et al., "Effect of coenzyme Q-10 therapy in patients with congestive heart failure; a long-term multicenter randomized study," *Clin Investig* 1993; 71(8 Suppl):S134-6.

7. Langsjoen, P., et al., "Long-term efficacy and effects of coenzyme Q-10 therapy for idiopathic dilated cardiomyopathy," *Am J. Cardiol* 1990; 65:521-523.

8. Langsjoen, P., et al., "Pronounced increase of survival of patients with cardiomyopathy when treated with coenzyme Q-10 and conventional therapy," *Int. J. Tissu Reac* 1990; 12:163-68.

9. Tran, M., et al., "Role of coenzyme Q-10 in clinical heart failure, angina, systolic hypertension." *Pharmacotherapy* 2001; 7:797-806.

10. Fugh-Berman, A., et al., "Herbs and dietary supplements in the prevention and treatment of cardiovascular disease," *Prev Cardiol* 2000; 3(1):24-32.

11. Puccjarelli, G., et al., "The clinical and hemodynamic effects of propionyl-l-carnitine in the treatment of congestive heart failure," *Clin Ther* 1992; 141(11):379-84.

12. Azuma, J., et al., "Double-blind randomized cross-over trial of taurine in congestive heart failure," *Curr Ther Res* 1983; 34(4):543-57.

13. Azuma, J., et al., "Therapeutic effect of taurine in congestive heart failure: A double-blind crossover trial," *Clin Cardiol* 1985; 8:276-82.

14. Schaffer, S., et al., "Interaction between the actions of taurine and angiotension II," *Amino Acids* 2000; 18(4):305-18.

15. Schmidt, U., et al., "Efficacy of the hawthorn (crataegus) preparation, LI 132 in 78 patients with chronic congestive heart failure defined as NYHA functional class II," *Phytomedicine* 1994; 1:17-24.

16. Cohen, N., et al., "Metabolic and clinical effects of oral magnesium supplementation in furosemide-treated patients with severe congestive heart failure," *Clin Cardiol* 2000; 23(6):433-36.

Chapter 15

1. Lukaczer, D. "Applied Endocrinology: Insulin Resistance and Chronic Disease," *Applying Functional Medicine in Clinical Practice.* Gig Harbor, WA: The Institute for Functional Medicine, 2002, p. 1-31.

2. Reaven, G., et al., "Pathophysiology of insulin resistance in human disease," *Physiological Reviews* 1995; 75(3):473-85.

3. Leclerre, C., et al., "Viscous guar gums lower glycemic responses after a solid meal: mode of action," *Am J. Clin Nutr* 1994; 59(Supp):776S.

4. Paolisso, G., et al., "Daily magnesium supplements improve glucose handling in elderly subjects," *Am J. Clin Nutr* 1992; 55:1161-67.

5. Paolisso, G., et al., "Pharmacologic doses of vitamin E improve insulin action in healthy subjects and non-insulin-dependent diabetic patients," *Am J. Clin Nutr* 1993; 57:650-56.

6. French, R., et al., "Role of vanadium in nutrition: metabolism essentiality and dietary considerations," *Life Sciences* 1992; 52:339-46.

7. McCarty, M., et al., "Complementary measures for promoting insulin sensitivity in skeletal muscle," *Med Hyotheses* 1998; 51:451-64.

8. Wascher, T., et al., "Effects of low-dose L-arginine in non-insulin diabetes mellitus: a potential role for nitric oxide," *Med Sci Res* 1993; 21:669-70.

9. Konrad, T., et al., "Alpha-lipoic acid treatment decreases serum lactate and pyruvate cones and improves glucose effectiveness in lean and obese patients with type 2 diabetes," *Diabetes Care* 1999; 22(2):280-87.

10. MacDonald, H., et al., "Conjugated linolenic acid and disease prevention: a review of current knowledge," J. Am Col Nutr 2000; 19(2):111S-118S.

11. Del Toma, E., et al., "Soluble and insoluble dietary fibre in diabetic diets," *Eur J. Clin Nutr* 1988; 42:313-19.

12. Galvan, A., et al., "Insulin decrease circulating vitamin E levels in humans," *Metabolism* 1996; 45(8):998-1003.

13. Verma, S., et al., "Nutritional factors that can favorably influence the glucose/insulin system: vanadium," *J. Am Coll Nutr* 1998; 17(1):11-18.

14. Boden, G., et al., "Effects of vanadyl sulfate on carbohydrate and lipid metabolism in patients with NIDDM," *Metab* 1996; 45(9):1130-35.

15. Fantus, I., et al., "Multifunctional actions of vanadium compounds on insulin signaling pathways: evidence for preferential enhancement of metabolic versus mitogenic effects," *Mol Cell Biochem* 1998; 182(1-2):109-119.

16. Lefebure, P., et al., "Improving the action of insulin," *Clin Invest Med* 1995; 18(4):340-347.

17. Ripa, S., et al., "Zinc and diabetes mellitus," *Minerva Med* 1995; 86(10):415-421.

18. Shamberger, R., et al., "The insulin-like effects of vanadium," J. Adv Med 1996; 9(2):121-131.

19. Preuss, H., et al., "The insulin system: influence of antioxidants," *J. Amer Coll Nutr* 1998; 17(2):101-02.

20. Seelig, M., et al., "Consequences of magnesium deficiency on the enhancement of stress reactions: preventive and therapeutic implications: a review," *J. Am Coll Nutr* 1994; 13(5):429-446.

21. Chausmer, A., et al., "Zinc, insulin and diabetes," *J. Amer Coll Nutr* 1998; 17(2):109-115.

22. Ibid., Crayhon, *Eating and Supplement Plans.*

23. Linday, L., et al., "Trivalent chromium and the diabetes prevention program," *Med Hypothesis* 1997; 49:47-49.

24. Luo, J., et al., "Dietary polyunsaturated (n-3) fatty acids improve adipocyte insulin action and glucose metabolism in insulin resistant rats: relation to membrane fatty acids,' *J. Nutr* 1996; 126:1951-58.

25. Paolisso, G., et al., "Daily magnesium supplements improve glucose handling in elderly subjects," *Am J. Clin Nutr* 1992; 55:1161-67.

26. Dominguy, L., et al., "Magnesium responsiveness to insulin and insulin-like growth factor I in erythrocytes from normotensive and hypertensive subjects," *J. Clin Endocrinol Metab* 1998; 83:4402-07.

27. Lukaczer, D., "Nutritional support for insulin resistance," *App Nutrit Sci Rep* 2001; p. 1-8.

28. Elamin A., et al., "Magnesium and insulin-dependent diabetes mellitus," *Diab Res Clin Pract* 1990; 10:203-09.

29. Anderson, R., et al., "Beneficial effects of chromium for people with type II diabetes," *Diabetes* 1996; 45:124A.

30. Anderson, R., et al., "Elevated intakes of supplemental chromium improve glucose and insulin variable in individuals with type 2 diabetes," *Diabetes* 1997; 46:1786-91.

31. Boden, G., et al., "Effects of vanadyl sulfate on carbohydrate and lipid metabolism in patients with non-insulin-dependent diabetes mellitus," *Metabol* 1996; 45(9):1130-35.

32. Macbash, M., et al., "Therapeutic evaluation of the effect of biotin on hyperglycemia in patients with non-insulin dependent diabetes mellitus," *J. Clin Biochem Nutr* 1993; 14:211-18.

33. Saltiel, A., et al., "Thiazolidinediones in the treatment of insulin resistance and type II diabetes," *Diabetes* 1996; 45:1661-69.

34. Jacob, S., et al., "Oral administration of RAC-alpha-lipoic modulates insulin sensitivity in patients with type-2 diabetes mellitus: a placebo-controlled pilot trial," *Free Radic Biol Med* 1999; 27(3-4):309-14.

35. Welinhinda, J., et al., "Effect of Moourdica charantia on the glucose tolerance in maturity onset diabetes," *J. Ethnopharmacol* 1986; 17:277-282.

36. Reaven, P. et al., "Dietary and pharmacologic regimens to reduce lipid peroxidation in non-insulin-dependent diabetes mellitus," *Am Clin Nutr* 1995; 62:1483S-89S.

37. Thompson, D., et al., "Micronutrients and antioxidants in the progression of diabetes," *Nutr Res* 1995; 15(9):1377-1410.

38. Jacob, S., et al. "Oral administration of race-alpha-lipoic acid modulates insulin sensitivity in patients with type-2 diabetes mellitus: a placebo-controlled pilot trial," *Free Rad Bio Med* 1999; 27(3/4):309-314.

39. Demattia, G., et al., "Reduction of oxidative stress by oral n-acetyl-L-cysteine treatment decreases plasma soluble vascular cell adhesion molecule-1 concentrations in non-obese, non-diplipidaemic, normotensive patients with non-insulin dependent diabetes," *Diabetologia* 1998; 41:1392-96.

40. Pieper, G., et al., "Oral administration of the antioxidant, n-acetyl cysteine, abrogates diabetes-induced endothelial dysfunction," *J. Cardiovascular Pharmacol* 1998; 32:101-105.

41. Samiec, P., et al., "Glutathione in human plasma: decline in association with aging, age-related macular degeneration, and diabetes," *Free Rad Biol Med* 1998; 24(5):699-704.

42. Bustamante, J., et al., "Alpha-lipoic acid in liver metabolism and disease," *Free Rad Biol Med* 1998; 24(6):1023-39.

43. Cunningham, J., et al., "Micronutrients as nutriceutical interventions in diabetes mellitus," *J. Am Coll Nutr* 1998; 17(1):7-10.

44. Takahashi, R., et al., "Evening primrose oil and fish oil in non-insulin-dependant diabetes," *Prostaglandins Leulcot Essent Fatty Acids* 1993; 49(2):569-71.

45. Anderson, R., et al., "Elevated intake of supplemental chromium improve glucose and insulin variables in individuals with type 2 diabetes," *Diabetes* 1997; 46(11):1786-91.

46. Malone, J., et al., "Diabetic cardiomyopathy and carnitine deficiency," *J. Diabetes Complications* 1999; 13(2):86-90.

47. Philipson, H., et al., "Dietary fibre in the diabetic diet: *ACTA Med Scand* 1983; 671(Suppl):91-93.

48. Cunningham, J., et al., "The glucose/insulin system and vitamin C: implications in IDDM," *J. Amer Coll Nutr* 1998; 17(2):105-08.

49. Horrobin, D., et al., "Essential fatty acids in the management of impaired nerve funcion in diabetes," *Diabetes* 1997; 46(Suppl2):S90-S93.

50. Gerbi, A., et al., "Neuroprotective effect of fish oil in diabetic neuropathy." *Lipids* 1999; 34(Suppl):93-94.

51. Salway, J., et al., "Effect of myo-inositol on peripheral-nerve function in diabetes," *Lancet* 1978; 1282-84.

52. Ibid., Packer, *The Antioxidant Miracle*, p. 45.

53. Morcos, M., et al., "Effect of alpha-lipoic acid on the progress of endothelial cell damage and albuminura in patients with diabetes mellitus: an exploratory study," *Diabet Res Clin Pract* 2001; 52:175-83.

54. Ziegler, D., et al., "Treatment of symptomatic diabetic peripheral neuropathy with the anti-oxidant alpha-lipoic acid. A 3 week multicenter randomized controlled trial (ALADIN study)," *Diabetologia* 1995; 38:1425-33.

55. Keen, H., et al., "Treatment of diabetic neuropathy with gama-linolenic acid," *Diabetes Care* 1993; 16(1):8-15.

56. Pacifici, L., et al., "Counter action on experimentally induced diabetic neuropathy by levocarnitine acetyl," *Int J. Clin Pharmacol Res* 1992; 12:231-36.

57. Quatraro, A., et al., "Acetyl-L-carnitine for symptomatic diabetic neuropathy," *Diabetologia* 1993; 38:123.

58. Okuda, Y., et al., "Long-term effects of eicosapentsenoic acid on diabetic peripheral neuropathy and serum lipids in patients with type II diabetes mellitus," *J. Diab Comp* 1996; 10:280-87.

59. Tatuncu, B., et al., "Reversal of defective nerve conduction with vitamin E supplementation in type II diabetics; a preliminary study," *Diabetes Care* 1998; 21:1915-18.

Chapter 16

1. Ibid., Sahley, *Anxiety Epidemic*, p. 65.

2. Hedaya, R., *The Antidepressant Survival Guide.* New York: Three Rivers Press, 2000, p. 198.

3. Ibid., Crayhon, *Eating and Supplement Plans.*

4. Linde, K. et al., "St John's wort for depression-an overview and meta-analysis of randomized clinical trials," *BMJ* 1996; 313:253-58.

5. Mehta, A., et al., "Pharmacologic effects of Withania somnifera root extract on GABA receptor complex," *Indian J. Med Res* 1991; 94:213-315.

6. Sakina, M., et al., "A psycho-neuropharmacological profile of Centella asiatica extract," *Fitoterrpin* 1990; LXI(4):291-96.

7. Ernst, E., et al., "Adverse effects profile of the herbal antidepressant St. John's wort (Hypercium perforatum L)," *Eur J. Clin Pharmacol* 1998; 54:589-94.

8. Bottiglieri, T., et al., "Folate, vitain B12, and neuropsychiatric disorders," *Nut Rev* 1996; 54(12):383-90.

9. Galland, L., "Neuroendocrine imbalance in patient care," *Functional Medicine Approaches to Endocrine Disturbances of Aging.* Gig Harbor, WA: The Functional Medicine Institute, 2001, p. 108.

10. Copper, A., et al., "Enhancement of the antidepressant action of fluoxetine by folic acid: a randomized placebo controlled trial," *J. Affective Dis* 2000; 60:121-30.

11. Tempesta, E., et al., "L-acetylcarnitine in depressed elderly subjects. A cross-over study vs. placebo," *Drugs Exp Clin Res* 1987; 13:417-23.

12. Garzya, G., et al., "Evaluation of the effects of L-acetyl carnitine on senile patients suffering from depression," *Drugs Exp Clin Res* 1990; 16:101-6.

13. Werbach, M., *Nutritonal Influences on Mental Illness: A Sourcebook of Clinical Research.* California: Third Line Press, Inc., 1991.

14. Penninx, B., et al., "Vitamin B12 deficiency and depression in physically disabled older women: epidemiological evidence from the women's health and aging study," *Am J. Psy* 2000; 157:715-21.

15. Edwards, R., et al. "Omega 3 polyunsaturated fatty acids levels in the diet and RBC membranes of depressed patients," *J. Affective Dis* 1998; 48:149-155.

16. Maes, M., et al., "Lowered omega 3 polyunsaturated fatty acids in serum phospholipids and cholestreyl esters of depressed patients," *Psychiatry Res* 1999; 85:275-291.

17. Hays, B., "Estrogen and depression," *Disorders of the Brain: Emerging Therapies in Complex Neurologic and Psychiatric Conditions.* Gig Harbor, WA: The Institute for Funcitonal Medicine, 2002, p. 282.

18. Birdsall, T., et al., "5-hydroxytrytophan: a clinically-effective serotonin precursor," *Alter Med Rev* 1998; 3(4):271-80.

Chapter 17

1. Head, K., et al., "Natural therapies for ocular disorders part two: cataracts and glaucoma," *Alt Med Rev* 2001; 6:141-66.

2. Wang, A., et al., "Use of carnosine as a natural anti-senesence drug from human beings," *Biochem* 2000; 65(7)869-71.

3. Quinn, P., et al., Carosine: its properties, functions and potential therapeutic applications," *Mol Aspects Med* 1992; 13(5):379-444.

4. Jacques, P., et al., "Long-term nutrient intake and early age-related nuclear lens opacities," *Arch Opath* 2001; 119(7):1009-19.

5. Cumming, R., et al., "Diet and cataract: the blue mountains eye study," *Opthal* 2000; 107(3):450-6.

6. Mares-Perlman, J., et al., "Vitamin supplement use and incident cataracts in a population-based study," *Arc Opthal* 2000; 118(11):1556-63.

7. "Preserving Clear Vision," *Life Extension* Feb. 2003; p. 30-7.

8. Robertson, J., et al., A possible role for vitamins C and E in cataract prevention," *Am J. Clin Nutr* 1991; 53:346S-351S.

9. Taylor, A., et al., "Long-term intake of vitamins and carotenoids and odds of early age-related cortical posterior subcapsular lens opacities," *Am J. Clin Nutr* 2002; 75(3):540-49.

10. Robertson, J., et al., "Vitamin E intake and risk of cataract in humans," *Ann NY Acad Sci* 1993; 372-82.

11. Olmedila, B., et al., "Serum status of carotenoids and tocopherols in patients with age-related cataracts: a case-control study," *J. Nutr Health Aging* 2002; 6(1):66-8.

12. Jacques, P., et al., "Long-term vitamin C supplement use: prevalence of early age-related lens opacities," *Am J. Clin Nutr* 1997; 66:911-16.

13. Varma, S., et al., "Scientific basis for medial therapy of cataracts by antioxidants," *Am J. Clin Nutr* 1991; 53:335S-345S.

14. Babizhayeo, M., et al., 'Efficacy of n-acetyl carnosine in the treatment of cataracts," *Drugs Research and Development* 2002; 3(2):87-103.

15. Giblin, F., et al., "Gluthione: a vital lens antioxidant," *J. Ocul Pharmacol Ther* 2000; 16(2):121-35.

16. Ibid., Crayhon, "Aging well in the 21st century," p. 27.

17. Seddon, J., et al., "Dietary carotenoids, vitamins A, C, and E., and advanced age-related macular degeneration,' eye disease case-control study group," *JAMA* 1994; 272(18):1413-20.

18. Winkler, B., et al., "Oxidative damage and age-related macular degeneration," *Mol Vis* 1999; 5:32.

19. Delcourt, C., et al., "Age-related macular degeneration and antioxidant status in the POLA study: POLA study Group, Pathologies Oculaires Liees a l'Age," *Arch Opth* 1999; 117(10):384-9.

20. Rose, M., et al., *Save Your Sight*. New York: Warner Books, 1998.

Chapter 18

1. Nies, K., et al., "Treatment of the fibromyalgia syndrome," *J. Musculoskel Med* 1992; 9(5):20-26.

2. Juhl, J., et al., "Fibrobyalgia and the serotonin pathway," *Altern Med Rev* 1998; 3:367-75.

3. Bralley, J., et al., "Treatment of chronic fatigue syndrome with specific amino acid supplementation," *J. App Nutr* 1994; 46(3):74-78.

4. Forsyth, L., et al., "Therapeutic effect of oral NADH on the symptoms of patients with chronic fatigue syndrome," *Ann Allergy Asthma Immunol* 1999; 82:185-191.

5. Abraham, G., et al., "Management of fibromyalgia: rationale for the use of magnesium and maleic acid," *J. Nutr Med* 1991; 3:49-59.

6. Behan, P., et al., "Effect of high doses of essential fatty acids on the post viral fatigue syndrome," *ACTA Neurologic Scand* 1990; 87(3):209-216.

7. Land, L., et al., "Antioxidative effective effective of ubiquinines on mitochondrial membranes," *Biochem J.* 1984; 222:463-66.

8. Packer, L., et al., "Alpha-lipoic acid as a biological antioxieant," *Free Rad Biol Med* 1995; 19(2):227-50.

9. Dalakas, M., et al., "Zidovadine-induced mitochondrial myopathy is associated with muscle carnitine deficiency and lipid storage," *Ann Neurol* 1994; 35(4):482-87.

10. Maddock., J., et al., "Biological properties of acetyl cysteine: assay development and pharmacokinetic studies," *Eur J. Respir Dis* 1980; 61(Suppl 111):52-58.

11. Rigden. S., et al., "Evaluation of the effect of a modified entero-hepatic resuscitation program in chronic fatigue syndrome patients," *J. Adv Med* 1998; 11(4):247-62.

12. Romano, T., et al., "Magnesium deficiency in fibromyalgia syndrome," *J. Nutr Med* 1994; 4:165-67.

13. Hawkes, K., *Breakthroughs in Managing Chronic Pain & Fibromyalgia*. Gig Harbor, WA: Metagenics Educational Programs, 2002.

14. Plioplys, A., et al., "Serum levels of carnitine in chronic fatigue syndrome: clinical correlates," *Neuropsycholbiol* 1995; 32:132-38.

15. Plioplys, A., et al., "Electron-microscopic investigation of muscle mitochondria in chronic fatigue syndrome," *Neuropsycholbiol* 1995; 32:175-81.

16. Ibid., Crayhon, *Eating and Supplement Plans*.

Chapter 19

1. ACE Seminar, "Understanding Fatigue: Addressing the Molecular Basis of Chronic Metabolic Disorders," 2001; p. 51.

2. Ibid., p. 51.

3. *The Importance of Detoxificaion*. Advanced Nutritional Publications, Inc. 2002.

Chapter 20

1. Johns, D., et al., "Mitochondrial DNA and disease," *NEJM* 1995; 333:638-44.

2. Ibid., Crayhon, *The Carnitine Miracle*, p. 61-64.

Chapter 21

1. Ibid., ACE Seminar, p. 56.

Chapter 22

1. Sult, T., *Functional Approaches to Resolving Chronic Health Disorders*. Gig Harbor WA: Metagenics Educational Programs, 2003.

2. Souba, W., et al., "The role of glutamine in maintaining a healthy gut and supporting the metabolic response to injury and infection," *J. Surgical Res* 1990; 48:383-91.

3. Lukaczer, D., "Gastroenterology, part II: gastrointerstinal disorders: clinical applications using the functional medicine perspective," *Applying Functional Medicine* in *Clincal Practice*. Gig Harbor WA: Institute for Functional Medicine, 2002.

4. Goldin, B., et al., "Health benefits of probiotics," *Br J. Nutr* 1998; 80(4):S203-7.

5. Bland, J., et al., "A medical food-supplemented detoxification program in the management of chronic health problems," *Aler Ther* 1995; 1(5):62-71.

Chapter 24

1. Ibid., Crayhon, *Level II Eating and Supplement Plans*.

2. Vogler, B., et al., "Feverfew as a preventive treatment for migraine: a systematic review," *Cephalalgia* 1998; 18(10):704-08.

3. Murphy, J., et al., "Randomised double-blind placebo-controlled trial of feverfew in migraine prevention," *Lancet* 1988; 2(8604):189-92.

4. Schoenen, J., et al., "Effectiveness of high-dose riboflavin in migraine prophylaxis. A randomized controlled trial," *Neurol* 1998; 50(2):466-70.

5. Thys-Jacobs, S., et al., "Alleviation of migraines with therapeutic vitamin D and calcium," *Headache* 1994; 34(10):590-2.

6. Thys-Jacobs, S., et al., "Vitamin E and calcium in menstrual migraine," *Headache* 1994; 34(9):544-6.

7. Thomas, J., et al., "Serum and erythrocyte magnesium concentrations and migraine," *Magnes Res* 1992; 5(2):127-30.

8. Gawel, M., et al., "The use of feverfew in the prophylaxis of migraine attacks," *Today's Ther Trends* 1995; 13(20):79-86.

9. McCaren, T., et al., "Amelioration of severe migraine by fish oil (n-3) fatty acids," *Am J. Clin Nutr* 1985; 41:874.

10. Ibid., Crayon, "Aging well in the 21st century," p. 27.

11. Rozen, T., et al., "Open-label trial of high-dose coenzyme Q-10 as a migraine preventive," *Cephalgia* 2001; 21:3880-81. Abstract P2-130.

Chapter 25

1. Ibid., Crayhon, *Level II Eating and Supplement Plans*.

2. Luper, S., et al., "A review of plants used in the treatment of liver disease: part I," *Alt Med Rev* 1998; 3(6):410-21.

3. Ibid., Packer, *The Antioxidant Miracle*, p. 31.

4. Stern, E., et al., "Two cases of hepatitis C treated with herbs and sypplements," *J. Alt Complemet Med* 1997; 3(1):77-82.

5. Niederau, C., et al., "Polyunsaturated phosphatidyl choline and interferon alpha for treatment of chronic hepatitis B and C: a multi-center, randomized, double-blind, placebo-controlled trial, Leich Study Group," *Hepatogastroenterology* 1998; 45(21):797-804.

Chapter 26

1. Ibid., Houston, *What Your Doctor May Not Tell You About Hypertension*, p. 2.

2. Ibid., Houston, *What Your Doctor May Not Tell You About Hypertension*, p. 40-42.

3. Ibid., Braverman, *Hyptertension and Nutrition*, p. 8-9.

4. Houston, M., "The role of vascular bioilogy, nutrition and nutraceuticals in the prevention and treatment of hypertension," *The Heart on Fire: Modifiable Factors Beyond Cholesterol*. Gig Harbor, WA: The Functional Medicine Institute, 2003, p. 81-84.

5. Ortiz, M., et al., "Antioxidants block angiotensin II—induced increase in blood pressure and endothelin," *Hyptertension* 2001; 38(3 pt. 2):655-59.

6. Ibid, Houston, *What Your Doctor May Not Tell You About Hypertension*.

7. Ibid., Braverman, *Hypertension and Nutrition*.

8. Sinatra, S., "Cutting edge technology in the prevention and treatment of cardiovascular disease: alternative interventions in treating cardiovascular disease," A4M Conference, 2003.

9. Silagy, C., et al., "A meta-analysis of the effect of garlic on blood pressure," *J. Hyperten* 1994; 12:463-68.

10. Digiesi, V., et al., "Coenzyme Q-10 in essential hypertension," *Mol Aspects Med* 1994; 15(Suppl):S257-63.

11. Borrello, G., et al., "The effects of magnesium oxide on mild essential hyptertension and quality of life," *Curr Ther Res* 1996; 57:767-74.

12. Sigh, R., et al., "Effects of hydrosoluble coenzyme Q-10 on blood pressures and insulin resistance in hypertensive patients with coronary artery disease," *Jour Human Hyper* 1999; 13:203-08.

13. Duffy, S., et al., "Treatment of hypertension with ascorbid acid," *Lancet* 1999; 356:2048-50.

14. Levison, P., et al., "Effects of n-3 fatty acids in essential hypertension," *Am J. Hypertens* 1990; 3:754-60.

15. Witteman, J., et al., "Reduction of blood pressure with oral magnesium supplementation in woman with mild to moderate hypertension," *Am J. Clin Nutr* 1994; 60:129-35.

16. Appel, L., et al., "Does supplementation with 'fish oil' reduce blood pressure? A meta-analysis of controlled clinical trials," *Arch Int Med* 1993; 153:1429-38.

17. Colin, P., et al., "Effect of dietary patterns on blood pressure control in hypertensive patients: results from the dietary approaches to stop hypertension (DASH) trial," *Am J. Hypertens* 2000; 13:949-55.

18. Sacks, F., et al., "Effects on blood pressure of reduced dietary sodium and the dietary approaches to stop hypertension (DASH) diet," *NEJM* 2001; 344(1):3-9.

19. Stevens, V., et al., "Long-term weight loss and change in blood pressure results of the trials of hypertension prevention, phase II," *Ann Int Med* 2001; 34:1-11.

20. Vollner, V., et. al., "Effects of diet and sodium intake on blood pressure: subgroup analysis of the DASH-Sodium trial," *Ann Int Med* 2001; 135:1019-28.

21. Ibid., Houston, *What Your Doctor May Not Tell You About Hypertension.*

22. Ibid., Sinatra, S., *Lower Your Blood Pressure in Eight Weeks.*

Chapter 27

1. Ibid., Schmidt, *Tired of Being Tired*, p. 18.

2. Ibid., Schmidt, *Tired of Being Tired*, p. 18-19.

3. Ibid., Crayhon, *Eating and Supplement Plans.*

4. Nobaek, S., et al., "Alteration of intestinal microflora is associated with reduction in abdominal bloating and pain in patients with IBS," *Am J. Gastroenterol* 2000; 95(5):1231-38.

5. Stenson, W., et al., "Dietary supplementation with fish oil in ulcerative colitis," *Ann Int Med* 1992; 116(8):607-14.

6. Belluzzi, A, et al., "Effect of an enteric coated fish-oil preparation or relapses in Crohn's disease," *NEJM* 1996; 334(24):1557-60.

7. Salomon, P., et al., "Treatment of ulcerative colitis with fish oil n-3-omega-fatty acid: an open trial," *J. Clin Gastro* 1990; 12(2):157-61.

8. Shoda, R., et al., "Therapeutic efficacy of n-3 polyunsaturated fatty acid in experimental Crohn's disease," *J. Gastroenter* 1995; 30 (suppl 8):98-101.

9. Gupta, Il, et al., "Effects of Boswellia serrata gum resin in patients with ulcerative colitis," *Eur J. Med Res* 1997; 2(1):37-43.

10. Liu, J., et al., "Enteric-coated peppermint-oil capsules in the treatment of irritable bowel syndrome: a prospective, randomized trial," *J. Gastroenterol* 1997; 32(6):765-68.

Chapter 28

1. Ibid., Rountree, *Immunotics*, p. 39-56.

2. Ibid., Crayhon, *Eating and Supplement Plans*.

3. Barringer, T., et al., "Effect of a multivitamin and mineral supplement on infection and quality of life. A randomized, double-blind, placebo-controlled trial," *Ann Int Med* 2003; 138(5):365-71.

4. Meydani, S., et al., "Vitamin E enhacement of T-cell-mediated function in healthy elderly: mechanism of action," *Nutr Rev* 1995; 53:552-58.

5. Meydani, S., et al., "Vitamin E supplementation and in vivo immune response in healthy elderly subjects," *JAMA* 1997; 277:1380-86.

6. Folkers, K., et al., "The activites of coenzyme Q-10 and vitamin B6 for immune responses," *Biochem Biophys Res Comm* 1993; 193(1):88-92.

7. DeSimone, C, et al., "The role of probiotics in modulation of the immune system in man and in animals," *In J. Immunother* 1993; IX(1):23-8.

8. Cunningham-Rundles, S., et al., "Nutrition and the immune system of the gut," *Nutrition* 1998; 14(7-8):573-79.

9. Chandra, R., et al., "Nutrition and the immune system: an introduction," *Am J. Clin Nutr* 1997; 66(2):460S-463S.

10. Harbige, L., et al., "Dietary n-6 and n-3 fatty acids in imunity and autoimmune disease," *Pro Nutr Soc* 1998; 57(4):555-62.

11. Thurnham, D., et al., "Micronutrients and immune function: some recent developments," *J. Clin Pathol* 1997; 50(11):887-91.

12. Burger, R., et al., "Echinacea-induced cytokine production by human macrophages," *Int J. Immunopharmacol* 1997; 19(7):371-79.

Chapter 29

1. Goldman, R., *Sleep: Essential for Optimal Health*. Chicago: American Academy of Anti-Aging Physicians, 2003, p. 19.

2. Ibid., Goldman, *Sleep: Essential for Optimal Health*, p. 1.

3. Ibid., Goldman, *Sleep: Essential for Optimal Health*, p. 1.

4. Ibid., Schmidt, *Tired of Being Tired*, p. 204-207.

5. Edling, C., et al., "Occupational exposure to organic solvents as a cause of sleep apnea," *Br J. Indust Med* 1993; 50:276-79.

6. Steiger, A., et al., "Effects of hormones on sleep," *Horm Res* 1998; 49(3-4):125-30.

7. Chesson, A., et al., "Current trends in the management of insomnia," *Emergency Med* April 2002, p. 11-18.

8. Ibid., Goldman, *Sleep: Essential for Optimal Health*.

9. Garfinkel, D., et al., "Improvement of sleep quality in elderly people by controlled-release melatonin," *Lancet* 1995; 346(8974):541-44.

10. Haimov, I., et al., "Melatonin replacement therapy of elderly insomnia," *Sleep* 1995; 18(7):598-603.

11. Hornyak, M., et al., "Magnesium therapy for periodic leg movements-related insomnia and restless legs syndrome: an open pilot study," *Sleep* 1998; 21:501-05.

12. James, S., et al., "Melatonin administration in insomnia," *Neuropsychopharm* 1990; 3(1):19-23.

12. Pastora, J., et al., "Flavonoids from lemon balm (Melissa officinalis L., Lamiaceae)," *Acta Pol Pharm* 2002; 59(2):139-43.

13. Speroni, E., et al., "Neuropharmacologicial activity of extracts from Passiflora incarnate," *Planta Med* 1988; 488-491.

Chapter 30

1. Ibid., Braverman, *Hypertension and Nutrition*, p. 179.

Chapter 31

1. Ibid., Roundtree, "Immune Dysfunction and Inflammation, Part II: Chronic Inflammatory Disorders," p. 28.

2. Albrecht, M., et al., "Therapies of toxic liver pathology with legalon," *J. Clin Med* 1992; 47:87-92a.

3. Ibid., Crayhon, *Eating and Supplement Plans.*

4. Goldin, B., et al., "Health benefits of probiotics," *Br J. Nutr* 1998; 80(4):S203-7.

5. Flora, K., et al., "Milk thistle (Silybum marianum) for the therapy of liver disease," *Am J. Gastroenterol* 1998; 93(2):139-43.

6. Luper, S., et al., "A review of plants used in the treatment of liver disease: part I," *Altern Med Rev* 1998;3(6):410-21.

Chapter 32

1. Ley, B., *Marvelous Memory Boosters.* Temecula, CA: BL Publications, 2000, p. 4.

2. Goldman, R., *Brain Fitness.* New York: Doubleday, 1999.

3. Ibid., Schmidt, *Brain Building*, p. 73.

4. Muldoon, M., et al., *Amer Jour Med* 2000; 108:538-546.

5. Ibid., Goldman, *Brain Fitness.*

6. Ibid., Perlmutter, *BrainRecovery.com*, p. 159.

7. Morris, M., et al., "Vitamin E and vitamin C supplement use and risk of incident Alzheimer's disease," *Alz Dis Assoc Disord* 1998; 12(3):121-6.

8. Seshadri, S., et al., "Plasma homocysteine as risk factor for dementia and Alzheimer's disease," *NEMJ* 2002; 346:476-83.

9. Kidd, P., et al., "A review of nutrients and botanicals in the integrative management of cognitive dysfunction," *Alter Med Rev* 1999; 4(3):144-61.

10. Crook, T., et al., "Effects of phosphatidylserine in age-associated memory impairment," *Neurology* 1991; 41(5):644-49.

11. Schreiber, S., et al., "An open trial of plant-source derived phosphatidylserine for treatment of age-related cognitive decline," *Isr J. Psychiatry Relat Sci* 2000; 37(4):302-07.

Chapter 33

1. Swank, R., et al., "MS in rural Norway: its geographic and occupational incidence in relation to nutrition," *NEJM* 1952; 246:721-28.

2. Swank, R., et al., "Effect of low saturated fat diet in early and late cases of MS," *Lancet* 1990; 336:37-39.

3. Swank, R., et al., "MS: the lipid relationship," *Am J. Clin Nutr* 1988; 48(6):1387-39.

4. Ghadrian, P., et al., "Nutritional factors in the aetiology of MS: A case-control study in Montreal Canada," *Int J. Epidmiol* 1998; 27(5):845-852.

5. Delanty, N., et al., "Antioxidant therapy in neurologic disease," *Arch Neruol* 2000; 57:1265-70.

6. Swank, R., et al., "Multiple sclerosis: twenty years on a low fat diet," *Arch Neurol* 1970; 23:460-74.

7. Laur, K., et al., "Diet and multiple sclerosis," *Neurology* 1997; 49(Suppl 2):S55-S61.

8. Rudick, R., et al., "Management of multiple sclerosis," *NEJM* 1997; 337(22):1604-67.

9. Ibid., Perlmutter, *BrainRecovery.com*.

10. Dworkin, R., et al., "Linoleic acid and multiple sclerosis: a reanalysis of three double-blind trials," *Neurology* 1984; 34:1441-45.

11. Reynolds, E., et al., "Multiple sclerosis and vitamin B12 metabolism," *Jour Neuroimmun* 1992; 40:225-30.

12. Nieves, J., et al., "High prevalence of vitamin D deficiency and reduced bone mass in multiple sclerosis," *Neurol* 1994; 44(9):1687-92.

13. Hayes, C., et al., "Vitamin D and multiple sclerosis," *Proc Soc Exp Biol Med* 1997; 216:121-27.

14. Nordvik, I., et al., "Effect of dietary advice and nn-3 supplementation in newly diagnosed multiple sclerosis patients," *Acta Neurol Scand* 2000; 102:143-49.

15. Perlmutter, D., "Multiple Sclerosis—functional approaches," *Townsend Letter For Doctors and Patients* Nov. 2003; #244.

Chapter 35

1. Gaby, A., *Preventing and Reversing Osteoporosis*. Rocklin, CA: Prima Publishing, 1994; p. 2.

2. Ibid., Gaby, *Preventing and Reversing Osteoporosis*, p. 4.

3. Coats, C., et al., "Negative effects of high protein diet," *Fam Prac Recert* 1990; 12(12):80-8.

4. Ibid., Gittleman, *Super Nutrition For Menopause*, p. 45.

5. Lloyd, T., et al., "Dietary caffeine intake and bone status of postmenopausal women," *Am J Clin Nutr* 1997; 65(6):1826-30.

6. Krall, E., et al., "Smoking increases bone loss and decreases intestinal calcium absorption," *J. Bone Miner Res* 1999; 14(2):215-20.

7. Melhus, H., et al., "Smoking, antioxidant vitamins, and the risk of hip fracture," *J. Bone Miner Res* 1999; 14(1):129-35.

8. Niewoehner, C., et al., "Steroid-induced osteoporosis. Are your asthmatic patients at risk? *Postgrad Med* 1999; 105(3):79-83, 87-88, 91.

9. Ibid., Crayhon, *Eating and Supplement Plans.*

10. Dimai, H., et al., "Daily oral magnesium supplementation suppresses bone turnover in young adult males," *J. Clin Endocrin Metab* 1998; 83(8):2742-48.

11. Sojka, J., et al., "Magnesium supplementation and osteoporosis," *Nutr Rev* 1995; 53(3):71-4.

12. Head, K., et al., "Ipriflavone: an important bone-building isoflavone," *Altern Med Rev* 1999; 4(1):10-22.

13. Kruger, M., et al., "Calcium, gamma-linolenic acid and eicosapentaenoic acid supplementation in senile osteoporosis," *Aging* (Milano) 1998; 10(5):385-94.

14. Dawson-Hughes, B., et al., "Effect of calcium and vitamin D supplementation in bone density in women and men 65 years of age or older," *NEJM* 1997; 337:670-76.

15. Agnusdei, D., et al., "Effects of ipriflavone on bone mass and calcium metabolism in postmenopausal osteoporosis," *Bone Mineral* 1992; 19(Suppl):S43-S48.

16. Reginster, Y., et al., "Ipriflavone: pharmacological properties and usefulness in postmenopausal osteoporosis," *Bone Mineral* 1993; 23:223-32.

17. Adami, S., et al., "Impriflavone prevents radical bone loss in postmenopausal woman with low bone mass over 2 years," *Osteoporosis Int* 1997; 7:119-26.

18. Ibid., Geramano, *Osteoporosis Solution*, p. 99-14.

19. Vermeer, C., et al., "Effects of vitamin K on bone mass and bone metabolism," *J. Nutr* 1996; 126(Supl 14):1187S-91S.

20. Tamatani, M., et al., "Decreased circulating levels of vitamin K and 25-OH vitamin D in osteopenic elderly men," *Metabol* 1999; 47(2):195-9.

21. Peris, P., et al., "Etiology and presenting symptoms in male osteoporosis," *Br. J. Rheumatol* 1995; 34(10):935-41.

22. Ooms, M., et al., "Prevention of bone loss by vitamin D supplementation in elderly women," *J. Clin Endocrinol Metabol* 1995; 80:1052-58.

Chapter 36

1. Ibid., Perlmutter, *BrainRecovery.com*.
2. Beal, M., et al., "Coenzyme Q-10 as a possible treatment for neurodegenerative diseases," *Free Rad Res* 2002; 36(4):455-60.
3. Shults, C., et al., "Effects of coenzyme Q-10 in early Parkinson's disease: evidence of slowing of the functional decline," *Arch Neurol* 2002; 59(10):1541-50.
4. Shults, C., et al., "A possible role of coenzyme Q-10 in the etiology and treatment of Parkinson's disease," *Biofactors* 2000; 9(2-4):267-72.
5. Sechi, G., et al., "Reduced glutathione in the treatment of early Parkinson's disease," *Prog Neuropsychopharmacol Biol Psychi* 1996; 20(7):1159-70.
6. Sato, Y., et al., "High prevalence of vitamin D deficiency and reduced bone mass in Parkinson's disease," *Neurol* 1997; 49(5):1273-78.
7. Fahn, S., et al., "A pilot trial of high-dose alpha-tocopherol and ascorbate in early Parkinson's disease," *Ann Neurol* 1992; 32(Suppl):S128-S132.
8. DeRijk, M., et al., "Dietary antioxidants and Parkinson's disease: The Rotterdam study," *Arch Neurol* 1997; 54:762-65.

Chapter 37

1. Ibid., Crayhon, *Level II Eating and Supplement Plans*.
2. Hansen, I., et al., "Gingival and leukocytic deficiencies of coenzyme Q-10 in patients with periodontal disease," *Res Commun Chem Pathol Pharmacol* 1976; 14(4):729-38.

Chapter 38

1. Ibid., Fillon, p. 82-86.
2. Ibid., Fillon, p. 32.
3. Leake, A., et al., "The effect of zinc on the 5 alpha-reducion of testosterone by the hyperplastic human prostate gland," *J. Steroid Biochem* 1984: 20(2):651-55.
4. Thomas, J., et al., "Diet, micronutrients, an the prostate gland," *Nutr Rev* 1999; 57(4):95-103.
5. Weisser, J., et al., "Effects of the sabal serrulata extract IDS 89 and its subfractions on 5 alpha-reductase activity in human benign prostatic hyperplasia," *Prostate* 1996; 28:300-06.
6. Wilt, T., et al., "Saw palmetto extracts for treatment of BPH," *JAMA* 1998; 280(18):1604-09.
7. Braeckman, J., et al., "The extract of serenoa repens in the treatment of BPH: a multicenter open study," *Ther Res* 1994; 55(7)776-85.
8. Liang, T., et al., "Inhibition of steroid 5 alpha-reductase by specific aliphatic unsaturated fatty acids," *Biochem J.* 1992; 285:557-62.

9. Niederprum, H., et al., "Testosterone 5 alpha-reductase inhibition by free fatty acids from sabal serrulata fruits," *Phytomedicine* 1994; 1:127-33.

10. Fotsis, T., et al., "Genistein, and dietary ingested isoflavonoid, inhibits cell proliferation and in vitro angiogenesis," *J. Nutr* 1995; 125:790S-797S.

11. Shippen, E., *The Testosterone Syndrome*. New York: M. Evans and Company, Inc., 1998, p. 211-212.

12. Ibid., Shippen, p. 49.

13. Ibid., Shippen, p. 50.

14. Ibid., Shippen, p. 212.

Chapter 39

1. Ibid., Crayhon, *Eating and Supplement Plans*.

2. Block, W., et al., "Modulation of inflammation and cytokine production by dietary (n-3) fatty acids," *J. Nutr* 1996; 126:1515-33.

3. Wright, S., et al., "Oral evening primrose seed oil improves atopic eczema," *Lancet* 1982; 2:1120.

4. Grattan, C., et al., "Essential-fatty-acid metabolites in plasma phospholipids in patients with ichthyosis vulgaris, acne vulgaris and psoriasis," *Clin Exp Dermatol* 1990; 15(3):174-6.

Chapter 40

1. Ames, B., "Micronutrient deficiencies: a major cause of DNA damage," *Metabolic Energy, Messenger Molecules, and Chronic Illness: The Functional Perspective*. Gig Harbor WA: The Functional Medicine, 2000, p. 196.

2. Murata, A., et al., "Smoking and vitamin C," *World Rev Nutr Bio* 1999; 64:31-57.

3. Scheetman, G., et al., "Ascorbic acid requirements for smokers: analysis of a populations survey," *Am J. Clin Nutr* 1991; 53:1466-70.

Chapter 41

1. Ibid., Schmidt, *Tired of Being Tired*, p. 120-122.

2. Heath, G., et al., "Exercise and the incidence of upper respiratory tract infections," *Med Sci Sports Ex* 1991; 23:152-57.

3. Sumida, S., et al., "Exercise-induced lipid peroxidation and leakage of enzymes before and after vitamin E supplementation," *Int. J. Biochem* 1989; 21:835.

4. Ryan, A., et al., "Over training in athletes: a roundtable," *Physician Sports Med* 1983; 11:93-100.

5. Shimomuray, M., et al., "Protective effects of coenzyme Q-10 on exercise-induced muscle injury," *Biochem Biophys Res Comm.* 1991; 176:349-55.

6. Colgan, M., *Optimum Sports Nutrition*. New York: Advanced Research Press, 1993, p. 247-61.

7. Ibid., p. 117.

8. Ibid., Crayhon, *Level II Eating and Supplement Plans.*

9. Balakrishnan, S., et al., "Exercise, depletion of antioxidants and antioxidant manipulation," *Cell Biochem Funct* 1998; 16(4):269-75.

10. Couzy, F., et al., "Zinc metabolism in the athlete: influence of training, nutrition, and other factors," *Int J. Sports Med* 1990; 263-266.

11. Pyke, S., et al., "Severe depletion in liver glutathione during physical exercise," *Biochem Biophys Res Comm* 1986; 139:926-31.

12. Antonio, J., et al., "Glutamine a potentially useful supplement for athletes," *Can J. App Physiol* 1999; 24:1-14.

13. Kelly, G., et al., "Sports nutrition: A review of selected nutritional supplements for endurance athletes," *Alt Med Rev* 1997; 2:282-95.

14. Lancha, A., et al., "Effect of aspartate, asparagine, and carnitine supplementation in the diet on metabolism of skeletal muscle during a moderate exercise," *Physiol Behav* 1995; 57(2):367-71.

15. Huertas, R., et al., "Respiratory chain enzymes in muscle of endurance athletes: effect of L-arginine," *Biochem Biophys Res Commun* 1992; 188(1):102-7.

16. Applegate, E. et al., "Effective nutritional ergogemic aids," *Int J. Sport Nutr* 1999; 9(2):229-39.

17. Campbell, W., et al., "Effects of resistance training and chromium picolinate on body composition and skeletal muscle in older men," *J. Appl Physiol* 1999; 86(1):29-39.

18. Clancy, S., et al., "Effects of chromium picolinate supplementation on body composition, strength, and urinary chromium loss in football players," *Int J. Sport Nutr* 1994; 4(2):142-53.

19. Bertelli, A., et al., "Carnitine and coenzyme Q-10: biochemical properties and functions, synergism, and complementary action," *Int J. Tissue React* 1990; 12(3):183-6.

20. Konig, D., et al., "Zinc, iron, and magnesium status in athletes-influence on the regulation of exercise-induced stress and immune function," *Exerc Immun Rev* 1998; 4:2-21.

21. Cordova, A., et al., "Behavior of zinc in physical exercise: a special reference to immunity and fatigue," *Neurosci Bebehav Rev* 1995; 19(3):439-45.

22. Mittleman, K., et al. "Branched-chain amino acids prolong exercise during heat stress in men and women," *Med Sci Sports Exerc* 1998; 30(1):83-91.

23. Elam, R., et al., "Effects of arginine and ornithine on strength, lean body mass and urinary hydroxyproline in adult males," *J. Sports Med Phys Fitness* 1989; 29(1):52-6.

24. Sen, C., et al., "Exercise-induced oxidative stress: glutathione supplementation and deficiency," *J. Appl Physiol* 1994; 77(5):2177-87.

25. Brilla, L., et al., "Effect of magnesium supplementation on strength training in humans," *J. Am Coll Nutr* 1992; 11(3):326-9.

26. Monteleone, P., et al., "Effects of phosphatidylserine on the neuroendo-crine response to physical stress in humans," *Neuroendocrinology* 1990; 52(3):243-8.

27. Bucci L., et al., "Selected herbals and human exercise performance," *Am J. Clin Nutr* 2000; 72(Suppl)624S-636S.

28. Ibid., Schmidt, *Tired of Being Tired*, p. 118-19.

Chapter 42

1. Ibid., Schmidt, *Tired of Being Tired*, p. 101.

2. Ibid., Schmidt, *Tired of Being Tired*, p. 101.

3. Fulder, S., et al., "Ginseng and the hypothalamic pituitary control of stress," *Am J. Chinese Med IX* (2):112-18.

4. Kelly, G., et al., "Nutritional and botanical interventions to assist with the adaption to stress," *Altern Med Rev* 1999; 4(4):249-65.

5. Gaffney, B., et al., "Panax ginseng and Eleutherococcus senticosus (Siberian ginseng) may exaggerate an already existing biphasic response to stress via inhibition of enzymes which limit the binding of stress hormones to their receptors." *Med Hypothesis* 2001; 56(5):567-72.

6. Rege, N., et al., "Adaptogenic properties of six Rasuyana herbs used in ayurvedic medicine," *Phytotherapy Res* 1999; 13:275-92.

7. Grandi, A., et al., "A comparative pharmacological investigation of ashwagandha and ginseng," *J. Ethnopharmacol* 1994; 44:131-35.

8. Darbinyan, V., et al., "Rhodiola rosea in stress induced fatigue—a double-blind crossover study of a standardized extract SHR-J with a repeated low dose regimen on the mental performance of healthy physicians during night duty," *Phytomed* 2000; 7(5):365-71.

9. Zhu, U., et al., "The scientific rediscovery of an ancient Chinese herbal medicine: Cordyceps sinensis," *J. Alt Comple Med* 1998; 4(3):289-03.

10. Tully, D., et al., "Modulation of steroid receptor-mediated gene expression by vitamin B6," *FASEB J.* 1994; 8:343-49.

11. Ibid., Crayhon, "Aging well in the 21st century," p. 24.

12. Ibid., Collins, p., 227.

13. Bland, J., "Normalizing HPA function," Nutritional Endocrinology: Breakthrough Approaches for Improving Adrenal and Thyroid Function. Gig Harbor, WA: The Functional Medicine Institute, 2002, p. 61-66.

Chapter 43

1. Ibid., Perlmutter, *BrianRecovery.com*, p.148.

2. Ibid., Crayhon, "Aging well in the 21st century," p.12.

Chapter 44

1. Ibid., Packer, *The Antioxidant Miracle*, p. 200.

Chapter 45

1. Ibid., Crayhon, "Aging well in the 21st century," p. 27.

2. Nezu, R., et al., "Role of zinc in surgical nutrition," *J. Nutr Sci Vitaminol* 1992; Spec:530-3.

3. Snyderman, C., et al., "Reduced post-operative infections with an immune-enhancing nutritional supplement," *Laryngoscope* 1999; 109(6):915-21.

4. Furukawa K., et al., "Effects of soybean oil emulsion and eicosapentaenoic acid on stress response and immune function after a severely stressful operation," *Ann Surg* 1999; 229(2):255-61.

5. Okeda, A., et al., "Zinc in clinical surgery—a research review," *Jpn J. Surg* 1990; 20(6):635-44.

6. Ibid., Crayhon, *Level II Eating and Supplement Plans*.

Chapter 46

1. Ibid., Smith, p. 47.

2. Nishiyama, S., et al., "Zinc supplementation alters thyroid hormone metabolism in disabled patients with zinc deficiency," *J. Am Coll Nutr* 1994; 13:62-7.

3. Meinhold, H., et al., "Effects of selenium and iodine deficiency on iodothyronine diodinases in brain thyroid and peripheral tissue," *JAMA* 1992; 19:8-12.

4. Berry, M., et al., "The role of selenium in thyroid hormone action," *Endocrine Rev* 1992; 13:207-20.

5. Kohrle, J., et al., "The deiodinase family: selenoenzymes regulating thyroid hormone availability and action," *Cell Mol Life Sci* 2000; 57:1853-63.

6. Brownstein, D., *Overcoming Thyroid Disorders*. West Bloomfield, MI: Medical Alternatives Press, 2002, p. 8.

7. Rouzier, N., "Thyroid replacement therapy," Longevity and Preventive Medicine Symposium. 2002, p. 2.

8. Pansini, F., et al., "Effect of the hormonal contraception on serum reverse triiodothyronine levels," *Gynecol Obstet Invest* 1987; 23:133.

9. Vliet, E., *Women Weight and Hormones*. New York: M. Evans & Company, 2001; p. 25.

10. Divi, R., et al., "Anti-thyroid isoflavones from soybean: isolation, characterization, and mechanism of action," *Biochem Pharmacol* 1997; 54:10, 1087-96.

11. Rachman, B., "Managing endocrine imbalance; autoimmune-induced thyroidopathy and chronic fatigue syndrome," *Functional Medicine Approaches to Endocrine Disturbances of Ageing*. Gig harbor, WA: The Institute For Functional Medicine, 2001, p. 226.

12. Shames, R., *Thyroid Power: 10 Steps to Total Health*. New York: HarperResource, 2001, p. 167.

13. Ibid., p. 47.

14. Ibid., p. 165.

15. Ibid., Crayhon, *Eating and Supplement Plans.*

16. Mano, T., et al., "Vitamin E and coenzyme Q-10 concentrations in the thyroid tissues of patients with various thyroid disorders," *Am J. Med Sci* 1998; 315(4):230-2.

17. Aihara, K., et al., "Zinc, copper, manganese, and selenium metabolism in thyroid disease," *Am J. Clin Nutr* 1984:40(1):26-35.

18. Maebashi, M., et al., "Urinary excretion of carnitine in patients with hyperthyroidism and hypothyroidism: augmentation by thyroid hormone," *Metabolism* 1977; 26(4):351-6.

Chapter 47

1. Diehmetal, C., et al., "Comparison of leg compression stocking and oral horse chestnut seed extract therapy in patients with chronic venous insufficiency," *Lancet* 1996; 292-94.

2. Ibid., Crayhon, "Aging well in the 21st century," p. 24.

3. Facino, R., et al., "Anti-elastase and anti-hyluronidase activities of saponins and sapogenins from Hedera helix, Aesculus hippocastanum, and Ruscus aculeatus: factors contributing to their efficacy in the treatment of venous insufficiency," *Arch Pharm* 1995; 328(10):720-24.

4. Siebert, U., et al., "Efficacy, routine effectiveness, and safety of horse chestnut seed extract in the treatment of chronic venous insufficiency. A meta-analysis of randomized controlled trials and large observational studies," *Ant Angiol* 2002; 21(4):305-15.

5. Pointel, J., et al., "Titrated extract of Centella asiatica (TECA) in the treatment of venous insufficiency of the lower limbs," *Angiology* 1987; 38(1Part 1):46-50.

6. Pittler, M., et al., "Horse-chestnut seed extract for chronic venous insufficiency. A criteria-based systemic review," *Arch Dermatol* 1998; 134:1356-60.

Chapter 48

1. Ibid., Crayhon, *Level II Eating and Supplement Plans.*

2. Ibid., Crayhon, *Level II Eating and Supplement Plans.*

Chapter 49

1. Ibid., Crayhon, "Aging well in the 21st century," p. 23.

2. Ibid., Crayhon, *Eating and Supplement Plans.*

3. Anderson, R., et al., "Effects of chromium on body composition and weight loss," *Nutr Rev* 1998; 56(9):266-70.

4. Blankson, H., et al., "Conjugated linoleic acid reduces body fat mass in overweight and obese humans," *J. Nutr* 2000; 130:2943-48.

Chapter 50

1. Ibid., Crayhon,, "Aging well in the 21st century," p. 26.

2. Bermond, P., et al., "Therapy of side effects of oral contraceptive agents with vitamin B6," *Acta Vitaminol Enzymol* 1982; 4(102):45-54.

3. Abraham, G., et al., "Nutrition and the premenstrual tension syndromes," *J. Appl Nutr* 1984; 36:103.

4. Pizzorno, J., "Natural hormone balance: assessing and forming treatment programs," *Functional Medicine Approaches to Endocrine Disturbances of Aging: Workshops.* Gig Harbor, WA: The Functional Medicine Institute, 2001, p. 197.

5. Williams, M., et al., Controlled trial of pyridoxine in the PMS," *J. Int Med Res* 1985; 13:194.

6. Facchinetti, F., et al., "Oral magnesium successfully relieves PMS mood changes," *Obstet Gynecol* 1991; 78:177-81.

7. Walker, A., et al., "Magnesium supplementation alleviates PMS symptoms of fluid retention," *J. Women's Health* 1998; 7:1157-65.

8. Ibid., Heller, *Applying the Essentials of Herbal Care.*

9. Lauritzen, C., et al., "Treatment of PMS with vitex agnus-castus controlled double-blind study vs. pyridoxine," *Photomedicine* 1997; 4(3):183-89.

10. Bendich, A., et al., "The potential for dietary supplements to reduce premenstrual syndrome (PMS) symptoms," *J. Am Col Nutr* 2000; 19(1); 3-12.

11. Sherwood, R., et al., "Magnesium and the premenstrual syndrome," *Am Clin Biochem* 1986; 23:667-70.

12. Kleijnen, J., et al., "Vitamin B6 in the treatment of the premenstrual syndrome—a review," *Br J. Obstetrics Gynaecol* 1990; 94:847-52.

13. Barr, W., et al., "Pyridoxine supplements in the PMS," *Practioner* 1984; 228:425-27.

14. Abrahm, G., et al., "Effect of vitamin B6 on PMS symptomatology in women with PMS syndromes. A double-blind, crossover study," *Infertility* 1980; 3(2):155-65.

15. London, R., et al., "Effect of nutritional supplement on premenstrual symptomatology in women with pre-menstrual syndrome: a double-blind longitudinal study," *J. Am Coll Nutr* 1991; 10(5):494-99.

16. Ibid., Crayhon, *Eating and Supplement Plans.*

17. Penland, J., et al., "Dietary calcium and manganese effects on menstrual cycle symptoms," Am J Obstet Gynecol 1993; 168(5):L1417-23.

18. Horrobin, D., et al., "The role of essential fatty acids and prostaglandins in the premenstrual syndrome," *J. Reprod Med* 1983:28(7):465-8.

19. Deutch, B., et al., "Menstrual discomfort in Danish women reduced by dietary supplements of omega-3-PUFA and B12 (fish oil or seal oil capsules)," *Nutr Res* 2000; 20:621-631.

20. Harel, Z., et al., "Supplementation with omega-3 polyunsaturated fatty acids in the management of dysmenorrhea in adolescents," Am J. *Obstet Gynecol* 1996; 174:1335-38.

21. Ibid., Smith, p. 82.

22. Murray, M., *The Healing Power of Herbs*. California: Prima Publications, 1995, p. 375.

23. Butterworth, C., et al., "Folate deficiency and cervical dysplasia," *JAMA* 1992; 267:528-33.

24. Bell, M., et al., "Place-controlled trial of indole-3-carbinol in the treatment of CIN," *Gynecol Oncol* 2000; 78:123-29.

25. Nestler, J., et al., "Ovulatory and metabolic syndrome and the effect of D-chiro-inositol in the PCOS," *NEJM* 1999; 340:1314-20.

26. Franks, S., et al., "Nutrition, insulin, and polycystic ovary syndrome," *Rev Reprod* 1996; 1(1):47-53.

27. Holte, J., et al., "Polycystic ovarian syndrome and insulin resistance: thrifty genes struggling with over-feeding and sedentary lifestyle?" *J. Endocrinol Invest* 1998; 21(9):589-601.

28. Hays, B., "Applied endocrinology: women's hormones and women's health," Applying Functional Medicine in Clinical Practice. Gig Harbor, WA: The Functional Medicine Institute, 2002, p. 5-7.

29. Ibid., Crayhon, "Aging well in the 21st century," p. 25.

Chapter 51

1. Quinn, P., et al., "Carnosine: its properties, functions and potential therapeutic application," *Mol Aspects Med* 1992; 13:379-444.

2. Roberts, P., et al., "Dietary peptides improve wound healing following surgery," *Nutrition* 1998; 14:266-69.

3. Vaxman, F., et al., "Can the wound healing process be improved by vitamin supplementaiton? Experimental study on humans," *Eur Surg Res* 1996; 28:306-14.

4. Vaxman, F., et al., "Effect of pantothenic acid and ascorbic acid supplementation on human skin wound healing process." A double-blind, prospective and randomized trial," *Eur Surg Res* 1995; 27:158-66.